THE LOVE HUNGER ACTION PLAN

Dr. Sharon Sneed

THOMAS NELSON PUBLISHERS
Nashville

D1384353

xx(4934889,2)

For general information about other Minirth-Meier Clinic branch offices, counseling services, educational resources and hospital programs, call toll free 1-800-545-1819.

National Headquarters: (214) 669-1733   1-800-229-3000.

Published in Nashville, Tennessee, by Thomas Nelson, Inc., and distributed in Canada by Lawson Falle, Ltd., Cambridge, Ontario.

Printed in the United States of America.

Scripture quotations marked NASB are from THE NEW AMERICAN STANDARD BIBLE, Copyright © 1960, 1962, 1963, 1967, 1971, 1972, 1973, 1975, 1977, by The Lockman Foundation and are used by permission.

Scripture quotations from the International Children's Bible, Copyright © 1988 by WORD, Inc., Dallas, TX.

Scripture quotations marked NKJV are from THE NEW KING JAMES VERSION. Copyright © 1979, 1980, 1982, Thomas Nelson, Inc., Publishers.

Library of Congress Cataloging-in-Publication Data

Sneed, Sharon, 1953–
    The love hunger action plan / Sharon Sneed.
      p.   cm.
    ISBN 0-8407-3461-1
    1. Reducing. 2. Compulsive eating—Treatment. I. Title.
RM222.2.S632 1992
613.2′5—dc20
                                           92–23652
                                           CIP

1 2 3 4 5 6 7 8 9 10 — 96 95 94 93 92

CONTENTS

Diary of a Counselor

Today is the day that all the fourth graders have their weights and heights checked in P.E. class. I wonder what I will weigh? It'll be a lot, I know. I think I am bigger than ever.

Good grief, it's hot in here. I can't concentrate on my work. What's Mrs. Martin talking about, anyway? English? Why did I wear all these heavy clothes? What time is it—maybe we'll have a fire drill instead of P.E. Maybe I could pretend that I'm sick. I wonder if I could fake a stomach-ache? Oh, God, why couldn't I have just been sick today? Then all my problems would be solved. I wonder if anyone else in class is worrying about this? Am I the only one who remembers that this is weight-check day?

Mrs. Peavis, the P.E. teacher, is nice. But I know she will call out everyone's weight and height in front of the whole class. Mine will be the highest, as usual. Probably even higher than Jack's weight—he's the tallest boy in class. Everyone will make fun and laugh at me. I just hate this. Please, God, get me out of here!

When I was a child, I always wondered if I was just born fat. And, for a few fretful years, each week was filled with some emotional trauma like the one above.

In case you don't know this already, being an overweight kid is rough, especially thirty years ago when we weren't making some attempts to accept each other as individuals. I remember being in eternal awe of Spanky in *The Little Rascals*. He managed to have a substantial weight problem and was still liked by all the neighborhood kids. I was ready to move into his house, his club, his neighborhood, his group.

I did have some good friends of my own. But at school I seemed to be a magnet for derogatory names from merciless classmates, mainly of the male gender. Shopping, too, was always a problem; I can remember having to squeeze into adult clothes that were then altered for my otherwise childlike stature. It just didn't seem fair. My friends seemed to eat what they wanted and never thought anything of it. Why did I have this problem?

I knew I was a smart little kid, and that helped some. I remember when we began algebra, everyone wanted to be my friend—or at least be close enough to see the answers on my paper. But soon everyone caught on to the new assignment, and their interest in me quickly disappeared.

Fourth grade really was the toughest time of my whole life from a child's perspective. I had a pudgy teacher named Mrs. Martin who reveled in making fun of my thirty-pound weight problem in front of the whole class. I just laughed with the rest of the kids, but it really cut to the quick, and then some. Even though I had a few good friends and a very supportive mother, it still smarted when I was chosen dead last in any kind of team or paired activity.

In those days, doctors told parents of overweight children, "They'll grow out of it." (Research does not support this—but that is another story.) Fortunately, I did slim down in junior high, and by high school I was a normal weight. But this was no accident or bit of natural evolution. I took up baton twirling, which eventually led me into about one hour of aerobic activity per day and gave me the emotional motivation to look good in my majorette costume.

I also decided to take dieting into my own hands. My typical teenage diet-day menu went something like this: nothing for breakfast, a hamburger without the bun for lunch, and a small steak and sliced tomatoes for dinner. (We were enamored with "no-carb" diets in the early seventies.) Then to balance this austere menu, I would have a dozen Little Debbie® something-or-others on the weekends. This continual cycle of binging and starving was a mainstay in the way I controlled my weight.

In college I gained only ten pounds over my high-school weight. This was no doubt due to a decrease in exercise and overall activity (all that studying, you know). I was twenty-one when I married, and I experienced another ten-pound gain when I discovered that I could actually make cakes, cookies, brownies, and other amazing culinary delights.

In 1975, when my husband, David, and I began our life together, the necessity for aerobics and lowfat eating was not a major social issue. Nor was it an issue for me personally. (I keep wondering what they discussed on talk shows in those days.) My husband was in medical school and I was in graduate school; and since we studied every waking moment, exercise was not exactly a top priority. Besides, food was the only reward we could afford. I know now that I had to learn food management.

LEARN MANAGEMENT, NOT ABSTINENCE

What's the first thing you want to do when you're told not to do something? Do it, of course! Human nature demands that you fight against any barriers that block your path. You don't know if the alternatives are good or bad, and you don't really care. All you know is that when someone gives you a resounding no, the hair on the back of your neck stiffens and rebellion is in your heart.

Yet, when a new weight-loss or healthy lifestyle program is begun, some sort of discipline must be established. Unfortunately, we tend to think of the word *discipline* in a negative way. Somehow we suspect that this new structure is going to muscle in on our fun. We innately want the freedom to do anything and everything our heart desires.

The discipline we've received in the past can actually affect how we accept boundaries now. What role did discipline play in your growing up years? Were you overdisciplined, to the point that there was no leeway for personal decision making? Or were there so few rules that now it is difficult to accept any form of regimentation?

The word *discipline* actually has two different connotations. The negative connotation gives us a sense of being chastised, corrected, and punished. Perhaps it takes us back to a feeling of shame or embarrassment. However, the positive connotation views discipline as control and moderation, as taking care of yourself.

Being the mother of three children, I have no doubt that discipline is absolutely necessary for healthy living. We are not born disciplined. We come into this world as self-seeking little creatures looking for our every whimsical desire to be met. We are taught discipline and hopefully we internalize it along the way.

If we have always thought of discipline as negative, we tend to rebel against dietary restrictions even if they are reasonable. These dietary boundaries become red flags, a jail to keep us from the freedom we desire. Or maybe we exist now in an overly restrictive environment, one in which we feel little freedom. So when we perceive yet one more boundary in our lives, we feel threatened and want to rebel, even though this is a boundary we would choose for ourselves.

Do diets make you feel boxed in or penned up, almost jailed? Do you feel like someone in a tight space desperately looking for some way out of this situation, like the drawing below?

You already know that the physiology of your body dictates either control of your eating to lose weight or loss of control to gain weight. Nonetheless, the discipline of dieting seems intolerable, so we just decide to quit playing that game. Or maybe we stay in the boundaries long enough to lose twenty pounds and then, in frustration, break out and say to ourselves, "I don't want any more boundaries in my life!" And the twenty-pound loss does not remain that way for long.

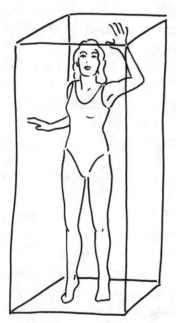

Don't set up dietary boundaries that are too limiting.

Now, I want you to compare this feeling with a new one. Imagine that the box—or diet—is enlarged. We can do this by adding a more reasonable amount of calories to our daily eating plans. (Very few people are able to stay on an extremely rigid diet plan for any length of time. When they fail, they are so discouraged that they even reject going on a more realistic program, which hardly seems like a diet at all.) We can even add amenities such as cooking instructions, a varied menu, and the ability to eat out. Then we put a door in the box so that we can actually go in and out without destroying the whole setup. It really is our choice to stay on—or go off—the diet. Yet we know that our food management plan is still waiting there for us when we return.

Finally, we realize that these walls or boundaries protect us from the onslaught of diseases related to overeating and obesity.

Can you see how a food management plan can make a profound difference in our ability to stay on a diet? Discipline can be good. It sets up boundaries that can protect. And they can promote a sense of safety and well-being. A food management plan can turn our ideas about self-indulgent eating around 180 degrees—food and fitness _____ ____ __ our friends; we don't need to hate or resent them. We _____ _____ __, with a caring discipline that

_____ ____ries as barriers that protect you.

LOVE HUNGER ACTION PLAN

After her weight began to return, a popular TV talk-show host and highly visible dieter said, "I will never weigh another piece of boiled chicken again!"[1] Well, Oprah, I don't blame you. And, if you had been my patient, you would not have had to do anything as legalistic and unappetizing as that in the first place.

You can actually eat a hamburger, fries, and lowfat ice cream sundae every night of the week (see recipes on pages 95, 225, and 223) and still lose weight, assuming you follow the suggested cooking methods and portion sizes! So, when I say to you, "Hey, lighten up!" it means be accountable and knowledgeable, not falsely legalistic.

Oprah Winfrey is like many Americans. They're fed up with off-and-on dieting. What they need is a sound maintenance program—a lifelong food management plan—that will help them keep the weight off once they've lost it.

The *Love Hunger Action Plan* is just that. Here is a ten-step plan to help those who have given up on diets begin again and to help successful dieters maintain their success for years—and even for life. These steps are summarized on pages xvi and xvii. As you glance through the steps you will see a new 25 percent-fat diet, which is a secret to long-term weight loss, and specific ways to fight cellulite deposits. You will see the specifics of a realistic food management plan and the psychological aspects of overeating—a new look at the love hunger we discussed in our previous books.

And you will see the amenities that enlarge your boundaries: optional food choices for eating out, special light fare for travelers, and an entire chapter of nutritious choices to some of your favorite, yet potentially unhealthy foods: "Instead of That . . . Try This!" Exercise is also a part of food management, and for the first time in the *Love Hunger* series we include a fully illustrated exercise program in Action Step 7. Finally, I give you 150 action tips toward permanent freedom from food addiction and weight gain problems.

But before we begin this ten-step process, let me ask that you approach this diet with four goals in mind.

FOUR GOALS FOR SUCCESSFUL
FOOD MANAGEMENT

1. Allow time for change in your life.

How many years have you struggled with your weight? Now ask yourself if it is rational to expect to solve this problem in a few months. In any recovery program, we must learn and relearn the same information. Sometimes we fail, but then we must pick ourselves up and walk again. We *can* hit the mark, but we must allow ourselves adequate time for success.

The rate of your weight loss is dependent upon how many pounds you have to lose. I once counseled with a 340-pound man who lost eighteen pounds his first week and fifty-four pounds in three months. For other people who have ten pounds to lose, a one-quarter pound loss is a real victory. Most men and women who have twenty to sixty pounds to lose will lose from one to three pounds per week. Don't sneer at one pound of fat. It is equivalent to four sticks of butter. Who wouldn't want to lose that?

Ultimately, you will lose what you lose. Individual bodies function differently. Don't worry about the weight loss. And don't compare your loss to someone else's. Instead, focus on your lifestyle changes, dietary changes, and exercise habits and just let nature take its course.

One further note: Do not check your weight more than one time per week or even one time per month. Daily weighing serves no purpose and is usually discouraging.

2. Educate yourself.

I have had scores of seasoned dieters tell me, "I know what to do. I just don't do it!" Many times these same would-be dieters don't know how to make a pizza that can be enjoyed by the whole family and still fit into a weight-loss program. Likewise, they don't know how to make a hamburger and french fries for about 400 calories (see pages 231 and 225), a 150-calorie grilled cheese sandwich (see page

230), or chips and dip (see page 227) that can be so good for you that you and your family may enjoy them every day. And who can really live without chocolate? Why not have a 150-calorie banana split (see page 223) a few nights per week instead of some lo-cal dessert with, shall we say, less pizzazz?

There is an art to eating well while you diet and even maintain your weight. But to do this you must be willing to

- Try new things
- Explore new ways of cooking and preparing foods
- Discard old recipes and some familiar ingredients—forever
- Have an open mind about "lighter" foods

Ultimately, you must educate yourself about nutrition, cooking, and fitness so that you can make your own decisions instead of depending on a book. You are the one at all those buffet parties, not me. Internalize the information in this and other credible diet books so that it is forever part of your own lifestyle.

3. Think food management rather than dieting legalism.

Many abstinence-type dieters I have counseled begin as black-and-white thinkers. They have been forced into this mode by the overly restrictive diets of the 1970s and 80s, which condemned food and the enjoyment of normal eating habits rather than helping you manage and make peace with food.

Two characteristics are almost universal to black-and-white thinkers. First, they feel that if the prescribed diet is not overwhelmingly restrictive (the abstinence type), it just can't work. *Moderation* is not in their vocabulary. Those of us who use this line of reasoning are continually setting ourselves up for failure, since this style of dieting will not carry over into normal living.

I have had phone calls from all over the country from panic-stricken dieters asking me about some minute detail concerning diet information in the first two *Love Hunger* books. These legalistic-type dieters usually have questions about how to calculate a small portion of a food exchange in various combination foods. For example, they might ask how to account for one tablespoon of chopped apple in a muffin (one bread exchange): "Would you count that small amount of apple as a fraction of a fruit exchange or just consider that it was unimportant and could be ignored?"

Though I certainly appreciate someone showing concern for the rules, we all know that one tablespoon of chopped apple does not make the difference in weight-loss success. It's the three cups of ice cream eaten at night when no one is looking that's the problem. Don't play games with yourself. Avoid legalistic concern over the small things, and confront the real issues head-on.

Second, black-and-white thinkers are either all good or all bad. The thought pattern goes something like this, "Gee, I've already blown my diet this morning with that stupid doughnut. Why did I eat that thing, anyway? Good grief, it was even stale. Well now, I guess it won't matter if I eat two more, plus blow it at lunch with my friends now that the day is shot, anyway. I'll start back on the diet tomorrow."

Come on. Doesn't that sound just a teeny-weeny bit familiar? When I was growing up, this philosophy reigned supreme as one of the major truisms in life. We were either really on the diet, or we were really off the diet. Another variation of this thought pattern is: "Calories eaten after I've already 'blown it' for the day (no matter how small the initial indiscretion) don't really count. Tomorrow I'll make up for all of this by starving myself." Right? Wrong, fellow dieters! Because you know and I know that tomorrow never comes.

Let's rebel against these restrictive thoughts. The truth is, abstinence from food—or even certain foods—is not required for weight loss; management of eating and lifestyle is. You will be able to eat many of your favorite foods, go out to dinner, and feel physically great while shedding that extra cargo.

So what if you have a few setbacks? Remember, we are not striving for perfection but overall management. According to the dictionary, a manager is "one who can cope with problems, direct, and bring order to a situation."

I have worked with hundreds of weight-loss patients over the last several years. Some do have this "I can't make a mistake on this diet or anything else" nature about them. They are often gregarious on the outside and about to crack on the inside. Perfectionism is stripping them of joy in almost every area of their lives. When holidays come, for example, and they eat more than they should, the audiotapes in their head tell them, "You blew it again, fatso. You'll never be able to do this or any other diet." Instead of falling prey to these thoughts, the dieter should applaud the past successes that have been made and look for constructive ways to be more fully prepared for the next holiday or special event.

So, the next time you fall off the wagon, don't lay in the rut and let the wheels roll over you. Unfortunately, perfectionism will often demand that you do just this in an attempt to punish and shame you. Remember, then, that perfectionism is unhealthy in any form—including dieting perfectionism. It always backfires.

4. Say No to Overindulgence.

One of the major obstacles to any program is learning to give up eating whatever you want, whenever you want. If you can just trust me on this one, you will soon see appropriate food choices and portion sizes become easier to manage after only a few months. And remember this, food compulsivity can take on two forms: not eating at all and eating too much.

For someone who has never used food as a friend, surrogate parent, or tranquilizer, this won't make sense. But the rest of us not only understand but identify with grieving for the loss of eating overindulgences as we would grieve for the loss of any good companion. For many of us, food was there when nothing or no one else was. It has become a reliable friend in good times and bad. It is affordable and always accessible. It never goes out of town or moves away. It is never too busy to nurture.

The grief process for giving up food as a friend and constant companion goes something like this.

You have just been told by your doctor that you must lose weight for health reasons. Or maybe you are just tired of buying a new wardrobe every year because of that extra ten-pound gain. But food has been a consistent companion for some time now. The

reality of not eating everything you want anytime you want it is set-
tling in. You are becoming uncomfortable. You're feeling like you
want to fight this thing. You resent God for making you into one of
those people who always need to diet. Maybe you even tell God
you hate Him for making you fat. You gnash your teeth and look for
any kind of magic that will get you out of having to diet the old-
fashioned way. The thought of food restriction and the "E" word
(exercise) turns your stomach. You feel as if you are two years old,
and you want to throw yourself on the floor just to kick, scream, and
cry until someone saves you from this terrible fate.

Friend, believe it or not, most dieters cross this same bridge of
tantrumish rebellion and true grievance many times. But the fact is,
you cannot continue a life of overeating and inactivity and expect to
remain slim or avoid weight gain. No magic pills or potions can save
you from the task before you. There are no quick fixes. In your
mind's quiet recesses of reason, you know this to be true and now
you must act upon it in an informed, patient, and positive way. Ultimately, the choice is yours.

There is no doubt in my mind that each person who reads this
has the ability to make the right choice. Be patient with yourself,
look for small successes, and compliment yourself. Love yourself by
choosing control.

The end of my own weight-loss story is this. I am several sizes
smaller than when I began my journey. I now control my weight,
and rarely do I gain even a few pounds. I am comfortable in knowing
I will never be model thin but am at a healthy and normal weight for
my body type. I continue to follow dietary guidelines put forth in all
the *Love Hunger* books.

Love Hunger Action Plan though, exemplifies how I really live
now. It is a dynamic, changing, accommodating, innovative eating
program that will work for and teach you. You have to learn to be
your own nutritionist. So study this book. Take it to heart. Make a
commitment today, and change your life forever.

From one dieter to another, I wish you well.

THE LOVE HUNGER ACTION PLAN

Action Step 1: Fight Fat

- The new 25 percent-fat diet (a secret of long-term weight loss as shown by new scientific discoveries)
- Ways to fight cellulite deposits

Action Step 2: Follow the New Love Hunger in Action Food Management Plan

- General guidelines for a successful weight-loss and maintenance program
- A detailed exchange diet, with expanded exchange lists
- Sample menus

Action Step 3: Develop New Eating Strategies

- Guidelines for grocery shopping
- Name brands you can buy at your local supermarket

Action Step 4: Instead of That . . . Try This!

- Alternatives for all your favorite restaurant foods, home cookin', trigger foods, and ingredients
- [Recipes for] Junk food and trigger food alternatives

Action Step 5: Set Your Mind upon Change

- Food as addiction and a philosophy
- Not forgiving those who cause your love hunger can destroy your diet
- Three excuses you need to put behind you
- Fulfilling your needs

Action Step 6: Adopt Winning Behaviors and Guidelines for Permanent Weight Loss

- The ground rules for eating out
- Specific foods to choose when eating out
- Special light fare suggestions for travelers
- Airline menu options

Action Step 7: Enjoy Fitness as Part of Your New Lifestyle

- A 45-minute, at-home circuit training program
- A fully illustrated exercise program

Action Step 8: Weight Loss Q & A: Know the Real Facts

- Answers to some of the most commonly asked questions in dieting
- Information on appetite control, natural foods, PMS and dieting, vitamin supplements, and much more

Action Step 9: 150 Action Tips for Permanent Weight Loss

- 150 quick-hitter suggestions to help keep you motivated and educated on the finer points of weight loss

Action Step 10: Be Prepared for Maintenance and Relapse

- The three most common reasons weight is regained
- The red flags of relapse
- The maintenance meal plan

Fight Fat

You can't win a battle when you don't know your enemy. In this action step we'll discover all we can about the fat cell and how it operates in your body. After all, none of us begins weight-loss programs because we are unhappy about our lean body mass (bone and muscle). Instead, we want to lose fat, and lose it permanently.

A SIGN OF THE TIMES

Until fifty years ago, starvation was a regular routine for some Westerners. If the crops were poor or pestilence caused a reduction in food supplies, then daily food fare might be on the light side. At the same time, work was more physical and not everyone had two cars in their garages. Walking, running, bicycling, or horseback riding almost everywhere was commonplace.

In those days, which were not so long ago, we burned more calories through activity and were occasionally required to use fuel stores for lack of immediate foodstuffs. The purpose of the fat cell was (and still is) to serve as an energy storehouse for those proverbial seven-year droughts and resulting famines. Each little cell holds a minute amount of concentrated fuel that you would have praised a few hundred years ago. Now, no longer fearing famine (at least in America), we often curse it.

Today one out of every two Americans wants to lose weight. And at least 25 percent need to lose weight for medical reasons. This constitutes an absolute epidemic of out-of-control fat cells. But fat cells have not changed over the last fifty years. So, what's the difference? First, it is fair to say that our definition of the "just right" body image has varied with the decades. The Twiggy generation needs to be considered Women's Enemy Number One. No one should have to fall below their normal weight in order to look attractive. But, because fashions and trends usually follow the newest fad, we all decided to lose twenty pounds when Twiggy became the "top model." Personally, you can give me those ol' Monroe and Grable days—putting that more realistic body type on an aerobic exercise program—and I think you'll have a "look" that everyone can live with.

To further prove this point, let me add something of a personal note. I grew up in the women's fashion business and had many wonderful times at the Dallas Apparel Mart. My mother was the owner and buyer for several ladies' apparel shops from the time I was ten years old. We frequently bought what were known as "samples." These were dresses that were made up to show buyers how a particular garment looked. They were also the ones worn by models in the showroom. The sample size (or model size) for clothing up until 1965 or so was size twelve. This would usually fit someone who was five-foot-five to five-foot-nine, weighing between 120 and 145 pounds. Hip measurements could go to thirty-seven inches and still easily fit into a size twelve garment. The cliché end-all measurements in those days were "36-24-36." Honestly, this more normal body type would not fly in today's fashion market where thirty-two-inch hips are expected. Sizes six and eight are today's sample sizes. And all the models who once weighed 135 pounds today feel compelled to weigh 120—even if they are five foot nine. They want us all to look like Barbie®!

I don't know how to advise you on this issue except to say that we should all attempt to find our own healthiest weight. Don't let faddish trends dictate the rules and discourage you from trying because the goal is not realistic. Very few people are ever going to look like Barbie®.

While our perception of the beautiful body was diminishing in size, our food supply was flourishing. Until you visit a foreign country, you don't realize how much emphasis is placed on food in the United States. And not just any food will do. The American palate has become accustomed to high fat, high sugar, or salt foods wrapped in cellophane, ready to be consumed at any time of the day or night. It's got to taste great, cost just a little, and be available on every street corner in every town of over two thousand inhabitants in order for a new edible product to make it in our marketplace.

The bottom line is this. We are an undisciplined society when it comes to our food choices and eating habits. And for those who have inherited the genetic capacity for obesity, these two factors of overindulgence and ready availability add up to what is often a lifelong struggle for weight control.

UNDERSTANDING THE FACTS ON FAT

What we commonly call body fat is known as "adipose tissue" in the medical community. This tissue is composed of millions of adipose cells, or, simply, fat cells, that are similar in structure to a balloon inside a balloon, except that they are microscopically small. The fat cells are not filled with air, however; they each contain a globule of fat, composed primarily of triglycerides. This small inner balloon forms the major part of any fat cell.

The fat globules inside the cells may have been made or synthesized by the fat cell. Or these cells are set up to accept fats that are floating around in the blood looking for a storage site.

Fat cells are very efficient. They basically just sit there until the body sends a biochemical message that there is a fuel deficit. They take very little energy to maintain. In fact, muscles in the resting state burn eight times more calories than the same amount of fat.

Now let's get specific. Fat tissue is actually between 60 and 90 percent triglyceride (something like oil, butter, beef fat, or lard). It contains six to eight calories per gram of tissue weight. If you consider that there are 454 grams per pound, then every pound of body fat stores roughly from 2,700 to 3,600 calories worth of energy that must be burned up in order to lose that pound of fat. If you were to have a five-hundred-calorie-per-day deficit, from either increased activity (roughly equivalent to walking five miles) or a decrease in food intake, you would lose one pound of fat every five to seven days.

For some of you, the thought of losing only one to one-and-one-half pounds of fat per week is enough to make you wince. Coming off of a decade of low carbohydrate diets that dehydrate you and make it seem as if you are losing weight quickly, you are accustomed to the belief that you can lose up to one pound per day. Folks, that is absolutely unphysiological and unrealistic, except perhaps for those few individuals who actually burn this many calories per day and do not replace these calories through eating. The only people who fall into that category are those who exercise all day or persons in excess of three hundred or more pounds who are concurrently on very low-calorie diets.

Most of us will lose about three to four pounds per week for the first two weeks, and then we will routinely lose one to two pounds per week. Even if you have lost only one-quarter of a pound, that is equivalent in size to a stick of butter. One whole pound is like losing a box of butter, and two pounds—well, just envision how much better your clothes would fit with four sticks of butter off each hip. Another plus for staying with your diet for the long haul is that, after being on the diet for more than twenty-one days, 90 percent of what you lose is fat tissue. Prior to that, some of the weight loss is attributable to water and protein loss.

The main areas of adipose tissue deposits are beneath the skin, between layers of muscle fibers, and around the internal organs. Anatomically, it is classified as a specialized connective tissue. That is, it helps connect the rest of the body. But, unlike tendons, this connective tissue can expand and decrease depending on caloric balance.

WHEN AND HOW DO FAT CELLS FORM IN THE BODY?

Fat cells are thought to be added only at specific times in your life. The accumulation of fat cells may actually begin *in utero*. If the woman gains an excess of weight during pregnancy (over thirty pounds), then it may be possible to add more fat cells to the developing baby. After this time, overfed infants may add fat cells in their first year of life. Adolescence and pregnancy are other stages in life when new fat cells are readily added.

Once a fat cell is part of your body, it can increase and decrease in size according to how large the fat droplet is that it contains. But even though you lose weight by decreasing each cell's size, the now deflated balloonlike cells remain a part of your body. The only way to get rid of the actual cells at this point is through surgical removal or a technique called liposuction.

Thus, body fat tissue may increase in size in two ways: by increasing the individual cell size (called hypertrophy) and increasing the actual number of cells (called hyperplasia). The typical fat cell in lean people weighs about 0.5 micrograms (μg) and can increase to an amount double that. After this size is reached, with continued positive energy balance (too many calories and not enough exercise) new fat cells can form. The number of total fat cells that can form is virtually unlimited. As stated above, once the fat cell is formed it does not turn into another type of cell or just disappear. It simply becomes smaller.

The normal American woman's body is composed of approximately 25 percent adipose tissue, which contains stored fat droplets and the supportive tissue to take care of these fat stores (including blood vessels and cellular membranes). Weighing 120 pounds, the typical woman thus has thirty pounds of this adipose tissue or body fat. If she gains forty pounds of weight, about thirty of those pounds will be actual fat globules inside fat cells. Her fat cells will in this case increase from an average of 0.5 μg to 1.0 μg. Above a thirty-pound weight gain this 120-pound woman would start making new fat cells.

The big moral to this story is whenever possible, stop weight gain before it occurs, especially large weight gain. Especially take note of this in your children. We can't assume that being overweight is something they will outgrow as they become older. Also, do not gain beyond thirty pounds while pregnant if at all possible, unless recommended otherwise by your physician.

If you are like me, however, and made every possible mistake in obesity prevention at almost every stage of life—there is still hope. With careful eating habits and a renewed interest in fat-burning physical activity, you can reach your goals. Everyone has the potential to lose weight, including you.

CELLULITE IS ANOTHER NAME FOR FAT

Cellulite is the common name given to the rippled look in the skin which is often present in the hip, stomach, and thigh region for many women (and some men), especially those who are overweight. Contrary to the sensational advice given in the national rag mags, cellulite is not caused by "toxins in your diet," "stressful lifestyles," or "not enough water." In fact, cellulite is nothing more exotic than a layer of fat below the skin. It is largely an inherited trait as to whether the appearance of fat will be rippled or smooth, and rippling seems to increase with age and the breakdown of connective tissue. Its appearance will decrease as your overall percent of body fat decreases and as you improve the tone of the underlying muscle.

The thing I want to save you from is all of the quack information concerning cellulite. No matter how many massages, body cremes, so-called "miracle" vitamin supplements, and other pseudoscientific information you may see about "getting rid of that unsightly cellulite," don't fall for it. These people are quick to gloss over the facts and just as quick to take your money. Cellulite can be controlled with weight loss, exercise, and toning. I know, I know, that's not as flashy as the twenty glasses of water a day and all the cantaloupe you can eat, but what makes sense to you?

Here's what you need to do to get rid of cellulite:

1. Achieve normal weight for your height through proper diet and exercise.
2. Keep up at least three sessions of aerobic exercise per week.
3. Make one of those weekly sessions a seventy- to ninety-minute moderate aerobic exercise (walking or bike riding) workout so that you can specifically work on fat-cell depletion. If you have no physical limitations, you should work toward walking six miles in ninety minutes.

4. Work on muscle toning three times per week. You may combine your aerobics and muscle toning by using the circuit training program in this book beginning on page 147.

THE HEALTH EFFECTS OF OBESITY

Well, there's more at stake here than our waistlines when we talk about total health. My typical weight-loss patient at the clinic is burdened with high cholesterol, high blood pressure, high triglycerides, and high taxes. No kidding. This person will usually have tried many diets, feels hopeless, and has now come in because their physician has basically told them to "lose weight or die."

After I calm their nerves and assure them that they will not die tomorrow, I explain that if they change their lifestyle they will have a real chance for the best health they have ever known. For many, dietary change, weight loss, and exercise can normalize elevated blood pressure, hyperlipidemias (too much cholesterol or too many triglycerides in the blood), and abnormal blood glucose levels (diabetes). It can also improve their immune system so that they are ill less often (even from the common cold) and have less chance of getting certain cancers. This goal is attainable and can be yours within a year. (Sorry, I can't do a thing about the taxes.)

Dr. Edward Bierman, Professor of Medicine at the University of Washington School of Medicine, has stated, "So profound is the relationship between obesity and disease that if the entire population were at optimal body weight, it is estimated that the coronary heart disease incidence could be reduced by 25 percent and congestive heart failure and [stroke] by 35 percent in the United States alone. [In fact, there might be] a 15 percent decline in mortality from better long-term weight management."[2]

To help reinforce what Dr. Bierman has stated, let's take one final look at the harm obesity brings and the help weight loss provides. Compare the following tables and see if there are health ramifications you have not previously considered.

Adverse Consequences of Obesity

Increased Mortality	Metabolic Consequences	Structural Consequences
Type II diabetes	Insulin resistance	Orthopedic impairment
Coronary heart disease	Hyperglycemia	Pulmonary difficulties
Stroke	Hypercholesterolemia	
	Hypertriglyceridemia	Surgical risk
Certain cancers	Low HDL cholesterol	
	Hypertension	
	Hyperuricemia	
	Gallbladder disease	

Reprinted by permission of Edwin L. Bierman, M.D., professor of Medicine, University of Washington School of Medicine, Seattle, WA.

Benefits of Weight Loss

- Improves coronary heart disease risk profile

- Normalizes triglyceride levels

- *Increases:*

    HDL cholesterol

    Glucose tolerance

    Insulin sensitivity

- *Decreases:*

    LDL cholesterol

    Need for antihyperlipidemic medications

    Blood pressure

    Need for glucose-lowering medications

Reprinted by permission of Edwin L. Bierman, M.D., professor of Medicine, University of Washington School of Medicine, Seattle, WA.

HOW TO DEPLETE YOUR FAT CELLS

We deplete our body's stores of fat by either using our muscles to burn extra energy or by restricting our caloric intake so that fat is burned to support bodily functions.

Muscles are actually designed to burn fat as their major fuel source when they are worked for long periods of time at a moderate pace. In the first twenty to forty minutes of aerobic exercise, your muscles will use immediate carbohydrate stores, which are stored within the muscles. This source of carbohydrate is called *glycogen*. It is considered your "fight or flight" fuel. It is ready at any time your muscles need an extra fuel spurt to do what your brain tells them to do.

When these stores are gone, the muscles turn to fat as the next fuel source. Thus, the longer you can exercise at a moderate pace beyond that half-hour mark, the more fat you will directly burn as fuel. This is something that can be a psychological self-boost when you are still in the questioning stage of an exercise program.

For example, perhaps most of your exercise efforts revolve around the thirty-minute walk you get in the middle of the day on your lunch hour. But on weekends you decide to walk six miles in an hour and a half. This exercise will really burn the fat. Just envision your muscles as incinerators throwing on "fat logs" that are going to just disappear out of your life. You can usually count on burning about eighty to a hundred calories of fat, or about one tablespoon of body fat, for every mile you walk after the first thirty to forty minutes.

For women, another issue is at stake. Some of the fat women add during pregnancy, which accumulates around the hip and thigh area, is somewhat metabolically protected. It was put there as a fat and energy source for the process of lactation (breast milk production). Some research has shown that this can be the most difficult type of fat to lose and that it can only be lost if the diet is accompanied by aerobic exercise.

Increased food intake is often mistakenly viewed as the chief cause of obesity, but reduced energy expenditure also contributes greatly to the problem. The components of energy expenditure (or the number of calories we burn up per day) include the resting metabolic rate (RMR), the thermic effect of food (or how much energy it takes to digest and utilize what you eat), and your level of physical activity. If your RMR is genetically low and you are very efficient in digesting foods you eat, the only way to manipulate your system is to eat fewer calories and to exercise more.

From experience I can say that many of my patients became sedentary in the past because it was so uncomfortable to exercise at their higher weight. It is something of a catch-22 and can begin as early as childhood. You don't exercise because your weight makes it uncomfortable to do so, thus, you become more obese and are even less likely to start an exercise program as the pounds add up.

Dr. Laura Pawlak stated in her book *Life Without Diets*, "Americans want a firm, youthful look. But how many are willing to spend the time and effort to achieve it? This 'do little, get lots' philosophy is incompatible with success." She goes on to say, "It's time to grow up and quit hoping for a weight-loss cure that allows you to remain lazy."[3]

I suppose that about sums it up. I just decided to let her use the bullhorn instead of me. But her words really are a challenge for all of us (me included!). We realize what we need to do but have yet to really determine to attempt these changes. And all the while our arteries fill with fatty deposits, our chances of cancer increase, our self-esteem decreases as the *Love Hunger* cycle spirals downward, and longevity is lost. Can we afford this? What's more important in your life than the next bag of chips and evening on the sofa? Think about it.

DON'T REFEED YOUR FAT CELLS

As we moderately restrict our calorie intake and increase our amount of activity each day, our fat cells will eventually diminish in size. It is very important that we do not refeed them, however. Only a few rules must be followed to avoid this refeeding process:

1. Don't binge eat—even on healthy, lowfat choices,
2. Avoid most high-fat foods; keep fat intake below 25 percent of the total calorie intake, and

3. Don't overdo complex carbohydrates and sugar unless you are actively involved in serious endurance sports.

When you have number one down, a topic discussed more in the previous *Love Hunger* books, numbers two and three are then the key to lifelong weight loss and maintenance. How many of your friends have lost several pounds only to gain them back again? Many of them lose the weight by using dietary supplements and then go back to making all their old food choices. If you go back to your old ways, you will also go back to your old weight. It is as simple as that.

There is no soft-pedaling this news—high-fat foods [like the ones listed on page 18] just can't be a part of your regular routine anymore. They must be given up, and appealing alternatives must be put in their place.

Imagine that you have already had the number of calories in a day necessary to maintain your weight. But you have been invited to a party that very evening. Once there, you eat a one-inch cube of cheddar cheese (in which 80 percent of the calories are fat) and two chips with a crab and cream cheese dip. Then you have a very small piece of chocolate fudge cake to top it off. All of the foods listed above are almost pure fat. The fat in these foods will go directly to storage if you have already had your calorie allotment for the day.

I was once at a morning coffee session where one woman was offered a cream cheese brownie. She responded, "Yes, in fact, I'll have one for each thigh." Though she really did not eat two brownies, her analogy was not far from the truth. The next time you are tempted to have something that is almost pure fat and is in addition to your normal intake, just imagine the fat content of that food product going directly to your hips or abdomen. Does this change the way you view the few seconds of oral sensation you feel when eating one of these foods?

DISCOVER WHERE HIDDEN FATS LURK

Hidden fats can occur in the least likely places, so you must become a food detective to discover where they lurk. They disguise themselves well in restaurants, grocery stores, and even in your own pantry. Knowledge followed by restraint is the key here.

What Is a 30 Percent-Fat Diet?

We hear this number bantered about by the American Heart Association, the American Cancer Association, the American Diabetic Association, and the American Dietetic Association. Everyone wants us to have less than 30 percent of our total caloric intake coming from fat. A few years ago the average intake of fat among Americans was closer to 40 percent and was even higher in many parts of the country.

To understand this concept, you must first know that there are several ways to report fat content. Let me relay a humorous story that may help you understand what I mean. Once when I was on the Minirth-Meier nationally broadcast radio program, I actually got what I must classify as "hate mail" from some ladies in Wisconsin. They were wives of cheese makers and dairymen. I had just explained on national radio that most natural brick cheeses have at least 80 percent of their total caloric content coming from fat. These farmers, however, had obtained information from local experts that their products contained a much lower percentage of fat, based on either the total volume or weight. They said, for example, that Wisconsin cheddar contained only 35 percent fat because out of one pound of cheese there was .35 pound of fat in the product. This has absolutely no bearing on the nutritional status of any food, however. The only thing that matters is what percentage of the calories in the cheese is fat calories. If the other method of measuring fat were used, then you could simply add water to a product and decrease its percentage of fat or fat content. Does that sound right to you?

To properly determine the percentage of calories coming from fat, you can use information on any food label in combination with the following equation:

$$\frac{\text{grams of fat} \times 900}{\text{calories}} = \% \text{ of calories as fat}$$

This simple equation is absolutely foolproof and is easy to use either in your head or with a pocket calculator. Now, here is an example:

```
NUTRITIONAL INFORMATION
PER PORTION
Portion Size (28g) ................. 1 Slice
Portions per package .................. 8
Calories ........................... 60
Protein g ........................... 4
Carbohydrates g .............. less than 1
Fat g ............................... 5
      Polyunsaturated fat g ............. 3
      Saturated fat g ................... 2

INGREDIENTS: Turkey, Water, Salt, Corn Syrup Solids,
   Flavorings, Milk Protein Hydrolysate, Sugar, Sodium
      Phosphate, Sodium Erythorbate, Sodium Nitrite.
```

The manufacturers and marketing executives of this particular turkey bologna would have us believe that this product is actually a healthy and wise choice. Emblazoned across the front of the package is the claim, "83% fat-free," making us believe that the product is only 17 percent fat. If that were really the case, then it would fall well below our criteria of a 25 percent upper limit. But they are basing that information on percent of fat by weight, while we now know that the only thing that matters is what percentage of the calories are fat. In truth, one slice of turkey bologna contains sixty calories and five grams of fat. According to our calculations, this would make turkey bologna 75 percent, not 17 percent fat as the manufacturer wants us to believe.

Now look at this food label from a Danish ham product.

```
          NUTRITION INFORMATION
             PER PORTION
        Portion Size: 1 Slice (21 grams)
          Portions per container: 8
Calories ........................... 25
Protein ........................ 4 grams
Carbohydrate ............. less than 1 gram
Fat ..................... less than 1 gram
Cholesterol ........... 10 mg (0.01 grams)
Sodium ............. 280 mg (0.28 grams)

   Ingredients: Ham (Cured with Water, Honey, Salt,
    Sugar, Sodium phosphates, Sodium erythorbate,
       Sodium nitrite), Caramel and Annatto coloring.
```

The ham has only 30 percent of the calories from fat (depending on the brand), while the turkey bologna has 75 percent of its calories from fat. The ham is clearly the better choice, and yet our mind-set tells us that poultry is always better than a pork product. This is where intelligent decision making comes into play. Keep all of these factors in mind the next time you visit your local supermarket. Arming yourself in this manner won't allow them to put one over on you.

(To obtain a clear picture of the general types of foods that contain greater than or less than 30 percent fat, see the chart on page 18.)

Deciphering Food Labels

In today's market nutrition labeling is required on packaged food only when some sort of nutritional claim or information is made about the product, or when there has been any vitamin, mineral, or protein fortification. The actual nutrition label (as seen above) must include calories, protein, carbohydrate, fat, sodium, iron, vitamin A and C, calcium, thiamine, riboflavin, and niacin. Other nutrients may be listed optionally. In the near future, new FDA guidelines will require that the amount of saturated fat, cholesterol, fiber, and calories coming from fat be listed. The *serving size* is totally up to the manufacturer. Often I see this manipulated to represent a nutritional profile that is more pleasing to the consumer. Some breakfast cereals reveal this marketing technique. If the cereal is too high in fat and calories, they simply reduce the serving size and reduce the amount of calories the purchaser sees. After all, who really measures the amount of cereal they eat in the morning?

Also, most labels design *ingredient lists* from greatest to least concentration by weight. A few exceptions to this rule include some staple items such as ketchup. However, it is my experience that most of the manufacturers list the ingredients on products such as these too.

Finally, we come to *health claims*. Since the 1980s these have become a major marketing tool for food manufacturers. We tend to believe anything in print, thinking that our government will protect us against health fraud. The problem is that the FDA can't keep up with all the claims, and this has left the work to be done through state agencies. It is a difficult battle; and unfortunately, as long as there are big profits to be made, there will be a motive for deception in this area as well.

I don't mean to imply that you should distrust all food labels. But when they make dramatic health claims, look at the facts to see if they are telling the truth.

Consider, for instance, that many peanut butter and vegetable shortening manufacturers claim their products contain "no cholesterol." This is true. What they don't tell you, though, is that the fat it does contain will cause you to form cholesterol within your own body. Or look at this label of light cream cheese.

```
NUTRITIONAL INFORMATION
PER SERVING
Serving Size ...................... 1 oz.
Servings per package .................. 8
Calories ........................... 70
Protein ............................ 3g
Carbohydrates ...................... 1g
Fat ................................ 6g
   Polyunsaturated ................. 0g
   Saturated ....................... 2g
Cholesterol ...................... 20mg
Sodium .......................... 115mg

INGREDIENTS: Pasterized Milk and Cream, Salt,
Cheese Culture, Stabilizers (Xanthan and/or
Carob Bean and/or Guar Gums)
```

The manufacturer implies that the product is so much lower in fat that it is a healthy and lowfat choice. However, if you use your percent of fat equation, you find that this so-called light cream cheese still gets over 65 percent of its calories from fat. That's more than a Hershey's chocolate bar!

Here's the bottom line. You must be wary of information that is boldly displayed on the front of the package and make sure you know what you are getting. Note the number of grams of fat and the calorie content per serving, then decide for yourself whether the product constitutes a good nutritional choice. Remember, according to our fat-fighting plan, a good nutritional choice is something that has 25 percent fat or less. If you know that you will be mixing this food with calories that are very low in fat (in the 5-10 percent range); then you may go up to 30 percent fat, and your 25 percent plan will average out.

There are a few exceptions to the rule. Almost all lowfat versions of mayonnaise, dressings, margarines, and other all-fat products still contain close to 100 percent fat. Though they have been diluted and modified, the basic calorie-containing components are still fat. In this case, you should look at the total number of calories you are consuming from this product. If you are using forty calories worth of salad dressing that contains three grams of fat, that hardly seems excessive in light of an entire meal. It is roughly equivalent to one teaspoon of butter or margarine. In fact, for every thirty-five calories worth of any kind of fat, you may figure it to be equivalent to one teaspoon of oil or butter.

THE 25 PERCENT FAT-FIGHTING DIET PLAN

I once heard a woman at the supermarket say, "I just don't know about all these lowfat diets. People need fat to be healthy too." They certainly do, but not to a great extent. This woman's argument is something akin to saying that Americans don't get enough sodium and should consider salting foods more heavily. In other words, it's ridiculous to think we don't get enough fat.

Diets have been suggested for heart patients all the way down to 10 percent of the calories coming from fat. Humans only require that 10 percent of the total caloric intake come from fat in order to maintain health. I suppose this is where they came up with that number. A 10-percent fat diet doesn't allow any frills. It is also painstakingly difficult to maintain. In this book, I am promoting a 25-percent-fat diet, which is at least 5 percent lower than many other weight-loss books. And, admittedly, it is a little higher than a few others. I base my recommendation on a new weight-loss study from Cornell University, which found that women on a diet which contained only 25 percent of the total caloric intake as fat lost weight with no other restrictions. That's it—no exercise, no calorie counting, no group therapy. I like this information. It is simple and to the point. Yet to cut out high-fat foods permanently is a big challenge.

For most packaged foodstuffs, combination foods, and frozen dinners, you should attempt to keep your food choices below that 25-percent-fat mark. Then, when you mix it with some fat-free foods plus a few all-fat foods (including any oil, margarine, and salad dressings), you will have something less or close to a diet containing 25 percent of its calories coming from fat.

Now check the following table to see which foods inherently have the least and greatest amounts of fat in their natural state. By "natural state," I mean that they have no butter, sauces, or gravies added. Rice means plain rice, not a commercial rice mix.

THE 25 PERCENT FAT-FIGHTING PLAN IN REVIEW

To follow a diet containing only 25 percent or less of the calories coming from fat:

- Choose combination foods that indicate a fat content of equal to or less than 25 percent fat according to the equation on page 12.
- On occasion you may choose foods of a higher percentage of fat if you will mix them with foods that contain very little fat.
- Avoid foods in the grocery store or in restaurants that may contain hidden fats.
- Choose a great proportion of your foods from the lowest fat categories below the 30 percent mark.

Foods and Fats

		% of Calories as Fat	Foods
UNDER 30% FAT	Choose most foods from this group.	0%	Egg white, rice (no added fat), most vegetables (excluding avocados), all fruits, sugar candy (jelly beans, gum, red hots, hard candies, candy corn, marshmallows, marshmallow creme, divinity (made without nuts and fat), most beverages, nonfat yogurt, nonfat specialty items.
		Less than 9%	Lean fish (cod, halibut, hake, redfish, orange roughy, Mahi Mahi), skimmed milk, nonfat yogurt, most flaked or nugget cereals that do not contain nuts or fats (check labels), most breads, corn tortillas, frozen yogurt desserts.
		9–19%	Light meat of turkey (no skin), shellfish (crab, oysters, lobster), flour tortillas, ice milk.
	Choose many from this group	19–29%	Light meat of chicken (no skin), 2% lowfat milk, lowfat cottage cheese, commercial rice mixes, many commercial frozen dinners specializing in lowfat food.
OVER 30% FAT	Choose a few foods from this group	30–39%	Round steak (no fat), dark meat of chicken or turkey (no skin), fatty fish (flounder, salmon, pompano), Danish ham, creamed cottage cheese, milk chocolate, most granolas, brownies, some cookies, cheesecake, muffins (unless made in more lowfat way), fruit pies, lean ground meat.
	Eat very infrequently from this group	40–49%	Most lean ground beef, beef liver, roasted and lean pork loin, sardines (no oil), cakes with frosting, biscuits, waffles, cream pies, pastries, ice cream.
		50–59%	Mozzarella part-skim cheese, parmesan cheese, chocolate bars with nuts, whole milk.
		60–69%	Whole egg, ricotta and mozzarella made from whole milk, Romano cheese, cheese sauce, regular-grind, ground beef.
		70–79%	Most brick cheese (including Cheddar, Swiss, etc.), peanuts, American cheese, ribs or rib roast, egg yolk.
		80–89%	Avocados, fresh coconut, sesame seeds, light cream cheese, most nuts (almonds, walnuts, pecans, etc.).
		90–95%	Most regular salad dressings (including Italian, French, Ranch, Thousand Island, Green Goddess, etc.), olives, cream cheese, macadamia nuts, sour cream, cream.
		100%	Meat fat, oils (all types), shortening, butter, margarine, oleo, nonstick cooking sprays.

Follow the New Love Hunger in Action Food Management Plan

It was one of those great fall days in the Midwest, just made for intramural sports. The familiar cool breeze brushed your cheek, the angle of the light told you that holidays were near, and the inexplicable smell of autumn was in the air.

On this particular Saturday the sixth-grade football championship game was about to begin. Spirits were running high as proud parents donned their teams' colors and craned their necks to pick out their very own young man. How was it possible that only a few years ago these same boys needed rocking, cuddling, and bedtime lullabies?

The whistle blew and the moment for the big game had arrived. The boys in blue ran onto the field as triumphant young warriors; and, in their helmets, padding, and uniforms, this bravado was accepted and encouraged. In the few minutes they had to warm up before the game, they tried to inconspicuously look back toward the bleachers, searching for the familiar faces of parents, grandparents, and family. These boys still needed the same intense reassurance they had always needed, just in more discreet ways. To a twelve year old, a distant wave from the stands is the equivalent of a kiss, cuddle, and "I love you" to a five year old.

Paul had played on the team for two years. He played well, was tall for his age, and was encouraged by the coaches to keep up his football efforts. Paul searched the weathered bleachers for any sign of his parents, but he knew in his heart that they were busy and would not be there. They never were. Yet hope lingered that today might be different. He kept thinking, "If only I were more of a star player, maybe they would come to my games." This effort to become a star and please others through his accomplishments became an overriding theme in Paul's life and affected him to a much greater degree than just intramural sports.

Paul was the third of four children growing up in a midwestern, Christian home of German heritage. His parents had the work ethic of two nations on their conscience, and the overflow from this intense sense of duty saturated their being. The family motto became *"Albeit macht das leben suess,"* which in English means "Work makes life sweet." As an adult, Paul later described his father as a workaholic who had very little time for anything other than work and church activities. Today, though Paul recognizes the importance of hard work, he finds his own "sweetness" in love, relationships, and joy of living daily for God instead of self. That's a far cry from the little boy who tried to win his father's favor on the football field. And the road to this new way of living was not always clear and smooth. Let's look at some of the discoveries he made about himself and how he managed recovery.

Paul was an intelligent and hard-working young man in his formative years. A great combination for achieving academic accolades—as he well did. He graduated from medical school, graduate school, and seminary before the age when many people are completing even their first degree. Somewhere, he managed to find time to marry and have three children.

This was a time of life when Paul could channel all of his compulsive tendencies into work instead of eating. In fact, he was very slim for his tall height and had even been teased about his thinness not so many years earlier. Once he even took protein pills in a last ditch effort to put on weight.

But by the age of thirty, compulsivity was slipping into other areas of his life. The will to please had become so intense that wear and tear was starting to show. At this time he was a professor at a university, counseling seminary students on weeknights, did free counseling in the ghetto on Saturdays, and taught in churches on Sundays. Amid this feverish schedule and will to succeed, Paul had also become many pounds overweight as a result of his newfound compulsive eating habits. A lot of those overachiever, "hero" types turn to food to relieve the constant pressure.

Paul was beginning to recognize the symptoms of burnout in himself but still wasn't sure what was driving him. As a good Christian man, he was under the impression that all his service and hard work was for God. But it pained him to see that his three great kids never seemed to think they had his full attention. When burnout became a serious issue (as invariably happens with workaholics), Paul called his friend and colleague, Dr. Frank Minirth. Oh, by the way, I neglected to mention that little Paul the football player grew up to be Dr. Paul Meier of the Minirth-Meier Clinics.

Frank tried to show Paul that he was still trying to achieve his earthly father's approval. Recognizing his own compulsive tendency to overwork and seek approval got Paul's full attention—though he wasn't quite sure he believed it all yet. Compulsivity had become a way of life, a good friend, and a comfort to Paul. And somehow he had felt justified in his incredibly busy schedule by using God's Holy Word. Matthew 11:30 says, "For My yoke is easy, and My load is light" (NASB). Today Paul admits, "It's easy to support an addiction you feel justified in having." But who was Paul really trying to please, his heavenly Father or his earthly father? Nowhere in the Bible does it say you must work at a breakneck, compulsive rate to please the Almighty.

Paul was starting to understand himself for the first time in his life. What were his motivations? What made him tick? This critical type of self-evaluation is the beginning of the healing process.

When the original *Love Hunger* team was put together, Paul provided tremendous insight because he was currently dealing with these issues himself. But healing hardly ever occurs rapidly or on cue. It takes time, dedication, understanding, and patience.

Paul determined that he would instigate a lifestyle program with the goal being the loss and maintenance of one pound per month. He adopted the *Love Hunger* diet, and over the next several years he managed to lose eighty pounds—and for the most part has kept it off! Yes, he grieved the loss of what was once one of his best friends—unlimited food in any amount and sort possible. No, the restrictions were not always easy. He would no longer stop by for snacks on the way home for dinner. But the change was permanent, complete, and heartfelt. Today he continues to make progress in more permanently engraining this new lifestyle in his daily living. Dr. Paul Meier is a case study in the success that comes with long-term food and health management. You can be too.

Dr. Meier's story is no different than that of a thousand other dieters. The difference is that his changes are strikingly complete. Statistics tell us that with older conventional diets (where only diet is discussed) you only have a 5 percent chance of succeeding. Obviously, I am not sugar-coating the situation. You have a tough job ahead of you. The only way to lose weight and keep it off is with a complete and long-term approach. Food, diet, and lifestyle management can be the successful keys that unlock the door of weight control for you just as they have for Dr. Paul Meier and myself.

CHOOSING A DIET

The Relaxed Approach

Choosing an eating plan, diet, or food management program is a personal issue. In my office I have just about as many diets as I have clients. Everyone has different needs, preferences, and abilities to stay within prescribed boundaries. Some people prefer an unstructured and laid-back approach, while others want every detail spelled out. As I tell you about two of my patients, decide which style suits you best.

Myra Jackson was and remains one of the happiest patients to ever walk through my door. She was such a joy to be with, I could scarcely justify charging her my professional fee. I never saw Myra without a smile on her face and something nice or funny to say. She was a divorced woman and had one son, aged five. She enjoyed her job at one of the microchip manufacturers here in Austin, Texas, and was heavily involved with her local Baptist church.

Myra had gained twenty-five pounds over the last five years since the birth of her son. At thirty-five, she had never been overweight before this time. She did not consider herself to be a compulsive overeater, though she enjoyed food and had a healthy appetite.

Needless to say, Myra Jackson was a busy woman. Full-time job, mothering, and church activities to boot. She told me at the beginning that she didn't want to be very hungry. (A little hunger was okay.) She also said that she was willing to make a thirty-minute commitment to walk at her lunch break, but she made no promises about exercise on the weekends. Expensive foods were not an option, nor did she have a lot of extra time for cooking. Finally, she was brave enough to just blurt out, "I really don't want to think about this much. I did Weight Watcher's before and couldn't stand all the adding up of foods eaten and not eaten . . . you know what I mean. What are we going to do about this? Do you have some ideas about dieting for someone like me, or am I a hopeless case?"

I responded as we laughed together, "Myra, of course there have to be rules to any diet plan. But if you are willing to lose a little bit slower and just 'soak up' some general principles for healthy living, well, I think we can make this work."

I designed a diet for Myra based on principles instead of menus or exchanges. She utilized all of the information on fat content and always avoided high-fat foods. There were certain things she would just not eat. She kept up two-and-a-half hours of walking per week and soon added a small workout with weights three times per week. She did this while watching the nighttime news. She was also provided with all the other material in this book and in general tried to be more careful about her weight, behaviors, and overall health habits.

It worked! Myra managed to lose all of her extra twenty-five pounds in four months and has at this writing kept the weight off. Losing a pound and a half per week may not sound flashy. On the other hand, little was required of Myra to do this. If one-and-a-half pounds of fat tissue contains at most 5400 calories (see page 3), then over the entire week Myra only had to burn up a few hundred extra calories per day (which she did by walking for thirty minutes per day, five days per week) and cut her daily calorie intake by about

500. So if she was normally taking in 1800 calories, she now took in 1300 calories.

Myra did not really concentrate on calories. Instead, we looked at her food diary to spot areas where she had eaten high-fat foods, inappropriate snacks, or large portions. As Myra's habits changed, so did her weight. Her maintenance diet was comprised of basically the same foods as her weight-loss diet, except in bigger portions. Sure, she added a few goodies once in awhile after the weight was off. But that, too, was under control.

If you would like to approach dieting as Myra has done, continue to read and take in all the information in the book. Then just operate off of head knowledge instead of setting up a formalized eating program. Adjust your normal diet and lifestyle so that it is uniquely you but reflects the good health habits put forward in this book.

The Structured Approach

James Eddington didn't want any part of this "laid-back" diet. He wanted me to tell him every detail of what, when, and how he should eat. James remarked, "I have always been overweight, Dr. Sneed. But I'm willing to give it another shot. I must have been on every diet in the book, and then some. I usually like to have you give me menus, exchanges, something where I pretty well know exactly what I am supposed to eat. Can you do that?"

"Sure," I replied, "but, at some point in the course you will have to make those decisions for yourself. When you are at a party, cafeteria, or at home a year from now, you will need to know enough to have actually become your own nutritionist. After we finish here, I only want to see you by chance, not as a repeat patient. My job from day one is to wean you off my information and instruction. In the meantime, though, we'll learn what it takes to lose weight. Okay?" James liked the approach and left with an exchange diet in hand.

Weight-Loss Principles for Everyone

There are many good eating and dieting programs, recipe books, and new slants on the whole area of healthy eating. I always encourage my clinic patients to look for new resources. Remember, we are not talking about some stiff program that says you always have to do it by the book, but a dynamic, ever-changing lifestyle that we are going to incorporate for now and always.

Either approach to dieting is fine. Take your choice: relaxed or structured. In either case you need all of the information in this book to make it work for you, permanently. Now, let's look at some basics that any food plan should include.

- Only 25 to 30 percent of the calories should come from fat. More than this will often result in fat-tissue increase, even if calorie intake is lowered. You can eat less fat than this. Anything above a 10-percent-fat diet is nutritionally adequate.
- It should include a wide variety of foods from all food groups. However, you may choose a vegetarian diet if you wish. But make sure you follow a diet that supplies all needed nutrients and complete protein sources. Do some extra reading on how to successfully and nutritionally be a vegetarian if this is your choice.
- A minimum of fifty grams each of carbohydrate and protein per day to assure that muscle tissue will not be broken down and used for fuel.
- A sufficient nutrient intake of important vitamins and minerals to promote optimal health.
- A food plan that meets your personal needs and considers preferences.
- A food plan that includes many bulky, low-calorie foods that can help fill up the empty spaces.

MORE SPECIFICS FOR A RELAXED WEIGHT-LOSS PLAN

Myra didn't want any hard-and-fast rules. You can diet this way, too, if you like. To reiterate this point, you may simply use the guidelines below if you are a fairly self-disciplined person who is happy to lose about a pound a week. You don't have to become involved with the more exacting exchange diet beginning on page 29 if the more general guidelines, plus new nutrition knowledge, seem adequate to help you revamp your own eating behaviors.

- Ninety percent of the time, eat only the "good for you foods" that have been discussed in the previous chapters and are listed in the exchange food lists.

- When you do have a food that is higher in fat and sugar, just enjoy it! Feeling guilty has no place in this diet. But when you are finished, know that it was a treat you have only once a month and that you can look forward to another next month.

- Double your intake of fresh or cooked vegetables and salads made from vegetables. Consume at least one cup of vegetables or salad at lunch and one-and-a-half cups at supper. (This is a minimum!) I have not had a successful dieter yet who refused vegetables.

- Women will not need more than four to six ounces of meat, fish, or poultry per day and men no more than eight ounces. A four-ounce portion is about the size of a hamburger patty.

- Drink at least eight medium-sized glasses of water or some other water-based beverage per day for a total of about 64 ounces. I prefer water with a twist of lemon or lime. This is now my standard beverage of choice in a restaurant.

- Reduce your overall intake of sweets, especially sweets that include large amounts of fat. Baked goods such as pies, cakes, cookies, and candy bars should be eaten very infrequently. One piece of standard, iced carrot cake is about five hundred calories. See page 221 for its alternative and other low-cal dessert ideas.

- Don't go out to eat more than three times per week. (Less would be better.)

- Become accustomed to taking your lunch and snack goodies to work. Use a small, insulated cooler to conveniently carry food and drink for the entire day. It can include sandwiches, diet colas, salads, fruit, and other great-tasting choices.

- Choose foods that crunch, foods that take a long time to eat, and foods that are on the "free" list with frequency.
- Avoid alcoholic beverages. Choose mineral water instead.
- Exercise at least four times per week for forty-five minutes each. The more you exercise, the quicker you will lose weight. Look at seven hours per week of strenuous exercise as a maximum.
- Avoid snacks that are more than 100 calories per item.
- Use behavior modification techniques to control portion sizes, second helpings, and other behaviorally related eating.
- Include skimmed milk or skimmed milk products at least twice daily if you are able to tolerate milk foods.
- Having a vague idea of how many calories you have eaten for the day is still okay, as long as you know that your food choices are generally low in fat, high in carbohydrate, and meet all other criteria listed above.

HOW MANY CALORIES DO I NEED?

You should base your new calorie intake upon what your ideal weight should be or what you would like to weigh. At least this is a good starting point. To determine your target weight, see the chart below. Ultimately, when you are within ten pounds of your target weight, you can determine the necessity for minor changes by how you look in the mirror.

After you have found your target weight, multiply that number by ten, and you will have a rough estimate of how many calories per day you should consume as you attempt to lose weight. For example if you were a woman who is five-foot-four who should weigh about 120 to 130 pounds, your caloric intake for a weight-loss diet should be about 1200 to 1300 calories per day. This should be comfortable and yet allow for a one to two pound per week loss.

Metropolitan Height and Weight Tables

Women

Height (without shoes)		SMALL FRAME	MEDIUM FRAME	LARGE FRAME
Feet	Inches	Weight in Pounds (without clothing)		
4	9	90–97	94–106	102–118
4	10	92–100	97–109	105–121
4	11	95–103	100–112	108–124
5	0	98–106	103–115	111–127
5	1	101–109	106–118	114–130
5	2	104–112	109–122	117–134
5	3	107–115	112–126	121–138
5	4	110–119	116–131	125–142
5	5	114–123	120–135	129–146
5	6	118–127	124–139	133–150
5	7	122–131	128–143	137–154
5	8	126–136	132–147	141–159
5	9	130–140	136–151	145–164
5	10	133–144	140–155	149–169

Men

Height (without shoes)		SMALL FRAME	MEDIUM FRAME	LARGE FRAME
Feet	Inches	Weight in Pounds (without clothing)		
5	1	105–113	111–122	119–134
5	2	108–116	114–126	122–137
5	3	111–119	117–129	125–141
5	4	114–122	120–132	128–145
5	5	117–126	123–136	131–149
5	6	121–130	127–140	135–154
5	7	125–134	131–145	140–159
5	8	129–138	135–149	144–163
5	9	133–143	139–153	148–167
5	10	137–147	143–158	152–172
5	11	141–151	147–163	157–177
6	0	145–155	151–173	166–187
6	1	149–160	155–173	166–187
6	2	153–164	160–178	171–192
6	3	157–168	165–183	175–197

Prepared by Metropolitan Life Insurance Company. Source of basic data: *Build and Blood Pressure Study*, 1959, Society of Actuaries and Association of Life Insurance Medical Directors of America. Used with permission.

THE EXCHANGE DIET
FOR THE STRUCTURED APPROACH

The exchange system may be familiar to many of you. In fact, we used a similar format in our previous books. The fact remains, no other system allows you to have more flexibility, be less hungry, get better nutrition, or lose fat faster than this one. Many health and weight-loss organizations utilize this system, including the American Diabetes Association, the American Dietetic Association, and Weight Watchers.

This is the approach to food planning that we used in the original *Love Hunger* book. In this book, however, we have greatly expanded the exchange lists to include many more foods and name brands. Additionally, the number of exchanges have been changed to reflect a new, lower fat diet. Now we are shooting for a 25 percent-fat diet, whereas before we were looking for a 30 percent-fat intake.

INSTRUCTIONS FOR AN EXCHANGE FOOD PLAN

James Eddington had returned to my office for his second visit. The previous week we had discussed generalities like exercise, commitment, and clearing the house of poor food choices. Today he was ready for structure.

I began explaining the program to James in this way: "James, you really can eat just about anything as long as you control the portion sizes. Even though this diet has structure, there is a lot of room for individual decision making. Look at these food exchange lists, James, (see pages 34–43 for your own copies of these lists). Foods appear on the same lists because they are nutritionally very similar."

James looked at the Starch/Bread list and asked, "Are you telling me that one slice of bread is the same as one-half cup of mashed potatoes or twenty Goldfish crackers?"

"That is essentially what I am saying," I replied. "Some foods have more nutritional value, some are higher in sodium; but when you talk about calories, carbohydrate, fat, and protein content, all the foods on an exchange list are similar. Here, look at this chart (see page 32), which summarizes the food exchange lists. You see, most starch exchanges have seventy calories in the quantities specified on the list and contribute all these wonderful nutrients, including all the B-vitamins."

"What about the other lists? Do they work the same way?" asked James.

"Yes, they do," I responded. "Look at the fruit list. We can see from our overview of the food exchanges that most of the fruits have about fifty calories, again, in the quantities specified. Now, look at the actual exchange list. From here you can see that a quarter cup of grape juice is the same calorie equivalent of one-and-a quarter cup of strawberries. Which would you rather have, James?"

"I've loved grape juice since I was a kid. But, good grief, one-quarter cup? That's make me feel like I'm at communion at church instead of having a snack. I'll stick with the strawberries," he said.

"That's where the decision making comes in," I said. "Exchange diets are all about getting the most taste and food for your daily allotment. It almost can become a game of sorts."

Sensing that he was ready for the next concept, I asked, "What would you do if your exchange allotment allowed you to have two or even three exchanges in one meal? Do you think they would all have to be the same food?"

James responded, "Since all the foods within an exchange list are nutritionally the same, I don't see why I would have to stick with just one thing. If I got two exchanges, I think I could double the amount of one item or choose one exchange of two different items on the same list."

"That is exactly right!" I said. "Now let's look at how we determine how many of these exchanges you will have per day. Look at the daily meal plans. They are divided into plans for those who consume milk and those who don't. Do you have a problem with milk allergies or lactose intolerance, James?"

"I don't think so," he said. "Maybe I'll fit into the group that takes milk. I really kind of like it."

I went on, "Now let's see how many calories you will need per day. Let's see, you should weigh about 180 pounds. So if we use our formula of eight to ten times your ideal weight for the number of calories per day that you should have, we come up with a 1440 to 1800 daily caloric intake. If you are willing to get some consistent exercise, I recommend that we split the difference and go with 1600 calories. What do you think?"

"That sounds good to me. I think I can commit to walking about ten miles per week," he said.

"Let's take a closer look at the number of exchanges you get in each food category when on the 1600 calorie diet including milk. You will actually be able to eat seven servings of starch per day. That's the same as seven pieces of bread, not that you just want bread. It just sounds like a lot of food to me. Look at this sample menu I have prepared for you (see page 45). Does this look like something you can survive on?" I asked.

"Survive? This looks like more food than I eat now! Are you sure about this? Can I really lose weight on this much food?" he asked quizzically.

"You can't believe how many patients tell me this," I said. "The difference is calorie density. From your food diary, I can tell that you have become accustomed to heavier foods that make it seem as if you eat very little. For instance, this little package of rye and cheese crackers you picked up at the gas station yesterday on your way home from work was three hundred calories worth of almost pure fat. You could have had a ham and cheese sandwich (light cheese and forty calorie bread), a cup of strawberries, and a glass of 1/2 percent milk for the same amount of calories and a lot less fat. I'm not even going to talk about other nutritional comparisons between the two meals."

I sensed I was on a roll with him and went on to say, "The key to weight loss is simple. You have to learn to get the most flavor, taste, and good food for your calories. Don't settle for junky, inadequate, poor-quality foods that really don't even taste good. Can I answer any more questions for you?"

"You have made it pretty clear already," he said. "I really think this is going to work. One further question, though. How do you suggest that I keep track of all the foods that I should eat during the day and how many I have had?"

"Here is a food diary you can use for that purpose. (See your copy on page 44.) Get several copies of this diary, and then take a new one with you each day. You might even plan the night before what you intend to eat the next day." And with that, James left my office until his next appointment.

INSTRUCTIONS FOR THE EXCHANGE DIET

1. There are six food exchange lists beginning on page 34. See the boxed information below to give you a general idea of how foods are divided into so-called exchange lists. Foods appear in the same list because they are nutritionally very similar. For example, a half cup serving of corn and one half of an English muffin are both starchy foods and have similar nutritional value. Thus, they are both on the starch list.

The Food Exchanges

Food Exchange List	Approximate Calorie Content per Exchange	Serving Size per Exchange	Major Nutrients Provided
Starch	70	1 slice or ½ cup	complex carbohydrates, B vitamins,
Meats	70	1–2 oz.	protein, iron, magnesium, chromium
Milk	80	8 oz.	calcium, phosphorous, protein
Low-cal Vegetables	10–30	Unlimited	folate, niacin, vitamins A, C, E, iron, calcium
Fruit	50	½ to 1 cup	vitamins A and C
Fat	40	1 teaspoon	essential fatty acids, vitamin E

2. Choose an appropriate calorie level using the previous charts in this chapter. Or you may simply do this by multiplying the weight you would like to achieve by ten or, for a little more restrictive diet, multiply by a factor of eight.

3. Find the calorie level most appropriate for you on the "Daily Meal Plan" chart on page 33. Follow across to determine how many exchanges from each group you can have for the day.

Daily Meal Plans

Total Daily Calories	Starches (1 serving)	Meats (1 oz.)	Skim Dairy Group (8 oz.)	Vegetables* (½–1 c.)	Fruits (1 serving)	Fats (1 serving)
For those who consume milk products:						
1000	4	5	2	3	3	2
1200	5	5	2	3	4	3
1400	6	6	2	4	4	4
1600	7	6	2	4	5	5
1800	9	6	2	4	6	6
2000	10	7	3	5	6	6
2400	13	7	3	6	8	7
For those who do not consume milk products:						
1000	5	5	0	3	4	2
1200	6	6	0	3	4	3
1400	7	7	0	4	5	4
1600	8	7	0	4	5	5
1800	9	8	0	5	6	6
2000	11	8	0	6	6	7
2400	14	8	0	8	8	7

*There is no quantity restriction on non-starchy vegetables as long as they do not contain added fat or sugar.

The Food Exchange Lists*

Starch/Bread List

(Each exchange contains approximately 70 calories)

Bread

Reduced calorie bread (40 calories/slice)	2 slices
White (including French and Italian)	1 slice
Whole wheat	1 slice
Rye or pumpernickel	1 slice
Raisin	1 slice
Bagel	½ small
English muffin	½
Pita	½, 6″ diameter
Hotdog bun	½
Hamburger bun	½
Matzo	1, 6″ square
Tortilla, corn	1, 6″ diameter
Tortilla, flour	¾, 8″ diameter
Melba toast	4
Bread sticks	3, 6″ long
Croutons, lowfat	¾ cup

Cereals

Bran cereals (such as All Bran, Bran Buds, etc.)	½ cup
Bran flakes	½ cup
Shredded Wheat	½ cup
Bran Chex, Ralston Purina	½ cup
Cheerios, General Mills	¾ cup
Cinnamon Toast Crunch	⅓ cup
Cocoa Puffs, General Mills	¾ cup
Corn Bran, Quaker	½ cup
Corn Chex, Ralston Purina	⅔ cup
Post Toasties, Post	⅔ cup
Cracklin' Bran, Kellogg's	¼ cup

Fibre One, General Mills	⅔ cup
Hearty Granola, Post	⅙ cup
Kix, General Mills	1 cup
Life, Quaker	½ cup
Nutri-grain, Kellogg's	½ cup
Puffed Rice, Quaker	¼ cup
Puffed Wheat, Quaker	¼ cup
Raisin Bran, Kellogg's	½ cup
Rice Chex, Ralston Purina	¾ cup
Rice Krispies, Kellogg's	⅝ cup
Special K, Kellogg's	¾ cup
Total, General Mills	¾ cup
Wheaties, General Mills	¾ cup
Wheat germ	2 Tbsp.
Cornmeal (dry)	2½ Tbsp.
Corn Grits, instant, Quaker	½ cup
Cream of Rice, cooked	½ cup
Cream of Wheat, cooked	½ cup
Malt-o-Meal, cooked	⅝ cup
Oatmeal, Quaker, cooked	½ cup
Ralston, Ralston Purina	½ cup

Crackers

Saltines, fat free (2″ square)	7
Saltines (2″ square)	5
Soda (2½ square)	3
Rye wafers	3
Melba Rounds	7
Oyster crackers	20
Rice cakes (2″ circle)	7
Pretzels	¾ oz.
Animal crackers	8
Arrowroot	3
Graham (2½″ square)	3
Vanilla wafers	5
Matzo	¾ oz.
Melba toast	5 slices
Crisp breads such as Wasa, Kavali	2–4 slices (¾ oz.)

Starchy Vegetables/Side Dishes/Ingredients

Cornmeal, dry	2½ Tbsp.
Flour, dry	2½ Tbsp.
Rice, grits, cooked	½ cup
Spaghetti, macaroni, noodles (no sauce)	½ cup
Beans, baked (no pork)	⅓ cup
Beans and peas, cooked, including kidney, white, split, pinto, black, and other varieties	⅓ cup
Peas, green, canned or frozen	½ cup
Lentils, cooked	⅓ cup
Potato, baked	1 small (3 oz.)
Potato, mashed (no added fat or gravy)	½ cup
Corn	½ cup
Corn on the cob (6 in. long)	1
Yam, sweet potato, plain	⅓ cup
Squash, winter (acorn, butternut)	1 cup
Popcorn (no fat added), popped	4 cups
Lima beans	½ cup

Starchy Foods Containing Fat

(Each exchange contains 100 calories per serving; count as one starch and one fat exchange.)

Pancake (4 in. across)	2
Waffle (4½ in. square)	1
Muffin, plain, medium	1
Biscuit (2½ in. across)	1
Corn bread (2″ cube)	1
Stuffing, bread (prepared)	⅓ cup
Taco shell (6″ across)	1
Whole wheat crackers, fat added, such as Triscuits and Wheat Thins	5
(see package)	4–8
Cracker, round butter type	6
French-fried potatoes, 2 to 3½″	10 (1½ oz.)

| Chow mein noodles | ½ cup |
| Potato chips | approx. ⅔ oz. or 7 chips |

Meat/Meat Substitutes
*(Each exchange contains about 70 calories and
3 grams of fat per serving.)*

Beef

Veal, tenderloin, round (bottom, top, all cuts), rump, sirloin, extra-lean ground round	1 oz.
Veal cutlets (ground or cubed, unbreaded)	1 oz.

Poultry

Meat of chicken, Cornish hen, turkey (without skin)	1 oz.

Pork

Leg (whole rump, center shank), ham, cooked, center slices	1 oz.
Canadian bacon, tenderloin	1 oz.

Lamb

Leg, rib, sirloin, loin (no visible fat)	1 oz.

Fish

Any fresh or frozen fish, canned salmon, tuna, mackerel, or other fish (water packed)	1½ oz.
Crab and lobster	¼ cup
Clams, oysters	1½ oz.
Scallops, shrimp, sardines (drained)	3
Tuna (water packed)	¼ cup
Tuna (canned in oil, drained)	¼ cup
Salmon (canned)	¼ cup
Herring (uncreamed or smoked)	1 oz.

Wild Game

Venison, rabbit, squirrel, pheasant, duck, goose (without skin)	1 oz.

Lunch Meat

95% fat free	1 oz.

Cheese

Lowfat cheese	1 oz.
Lowfat cottage cheese	1/3 cup
Grated Parmesan	2 Tbsp.
Ricotta, part-skim	1/4 cup
Mozzarella, part-skim	1 oz.

Dried Beans and Peas

Cooked, all varieties	1/2 cup

Eggs and Vegetarian Alternatives

Egg whites	6
Egg Beaters	1/2 cup
Whole egg (medium)	1
Tofu (2½" x 2¾" x 1")	3 oz.

Milk/Milk Products

(Each exchange contains about 90 calories.)

Skimmed or ½ of 1%	1 cup
Lowfat buttermilk	1 cup
Evaporated skimmed milk	1/2 cup
Dry nonfat milk	1/3 cup
Yogurt, plain nonfat	1 cup
Yogurt, light, no sugar, nonfat (fruit flavored)	1 cup
Cheese	
Lowfat cottage cheese	1/2 cup
Part-skim milk cheeses	1 oz.

Vegetables

(These may be eaten in unlimited quantities. They contain from 5 to 25 calories per ½ cup serving.)

Alfalfa sprouts	Chives	Onions
Artichoke	Collards	Parsley
Asparagus	Coriander	Pumpkin
Bamboo shoots	Cucumbers	Radish
Beans, green,	Dandelion greens	Rhubarb
wax, Italian	Eggplant	Sauerkraut
Bean sprouts	Endive	Shallots
Beets, beet greens	Green peppers	Spinach
Broccoli	Greens, mustard, turnip	Summer squash
Brussels sprouts	Kohlrabi	Tomatoes
Cabbage, all types	Leeks	Tomato/vegetable juice
Carrots	Lettuce, all types	Turnips
Cauliflower	Mushrooms	Water chestnuts
Celery	Mustard greens	Watercress
Chard	Okra	Zucchini

Fruit

(Each exchange contains about 60 calories per serving.)

Apple (raw, 2″)	1
Applesauce (unsweetened)	½ cup
Apricots (medium, raw)	4
Apricots (canned)	½ cup or 4 halves
Banana (9″)	½
Blackberries (raw)	¾ cup
Blueberries (raw)	¾ cup
Cantaloupe, whole	⅓ melon
cubed	1 cup
Cherries (large, raw)	12
Cherries (canned)	½ cup
Cranberries, no sugar	no limit
Currants	1 cup
Dates (medium)	2
Elderberries (raw)	½ cup

Figs	2
Fruit cocktail (canned, water pack)	3/4 cup
Grapefruit (med.)	1/2
Grapefruit segments	3/4 cup
Grapes	15
Honeydew melon (med.)	1/4
cubed	1 cup
Kiwi (large)	1
Limes	3
Loganberries	2/3 cup
Mandarin oranges	3/4 cup
Mango	1/2
Melon balls, cantaloupe, and honeydew	1 cup
Mulberries	1 cup
Nectarine (2 1/2″)	1
Orange (2 1/2″)	1
Papaya	1 cup
Peach (2 3/4″)	1
pieces	3/4 cup
Peaches (canned)	1/2 cup or 2 halves
Pear (large)	1/2
Pears (canned)	1/2 cup or 2 halves
Persimmon (med.)	2
Pineapple (raw)	3/4 cup
Pineapple (canned, juice pack)	3/4 cup
Plums (2″)	2
Pomegranate	1/2
Prunes	2
Raisins	2 Tbsp.
Raspberries	1 cup
Rhubarb	No limit
Strawberries	1 1/4 cup
Tangerine (med.)	1
Watermelon	1 1/4 cup

Dried Fruit

Apples	4 rings
Apricots	7 halves

Dates	2½
Prunes (med.)	3
Raisins	2 Tbsp.

Fruit Juice

Apple juice	½ cup
Cranberry juice cocktail	⅓ cup
Grape juice	⅓ cup
Grapefruit juice	½ cup
Orange juice	½ cup
Pineapple juice	½ cup
Prune juice	⅓ cup

Fats
(Each exchange contains about 40 calories.)

Avocado (med.)	⅛
Bacon	1 slice
Butter	1 tsp.
Chitterlings	½ oz.
Coconut, shredded	2 Tbsp.
Cream (light)	2 Tbsp.
Cream (sour)	2 Tbsp.
Cream (heavy)	1 Tbsp.
Cream cheese	1 Tbsp.
Margarine	1 tsp.
Margarine (diet)	1 Tbsp.
Mayonnaise	1 tsp.
Mayonnaise (diet)	1 Tbsp.
Oil, corn	1 tsp.
Oil, olive	1 tsp.
Oil, safflower, soybean, peanut	1 tsp.
Olives (small)	10
Salad dressings	1 Tbsp.
Salad dressings, light	1 Tbsp.
Salt pork	¼ oz.

Nuts

Almonds (dry)	6
Cashews (dry)	1 Tbsp.
Pecans	4 halves
Peanuts (small)	20
Walnuts	2
Sunflower seeds	1 Tbsp.
Pumpkin seeds	2 tsp.

Free Foods

(These may be eaten in unlimited quantities.)

Any vegetables from the list on page 39
Sugar-free jello
Condiments: mustard, picante sauce

Vinegar, lemon juice
Sugar-free drinks
Sugar-free chewing gum
Sugar-free popsicles

Herbs
Sugar-free candy
Bouillon, de-fatted food stock

Fast Foods

(Calorie levels listed at the end of this chapter)

Fried chicken fillet sandwich	3 bread, 1½ meat, 4 fat
Grilled chicken sandwich	2 bread, 3 meat, 1 fat
Hamburger (large)	4 bread, 3½ meat, 2 fat
Cheeseburger (large)	2 bread, 4 meat, 3 fat
Cheeseburger (average)	2 bread, 2½ meat, 1 fat
Fish sandwich (fried)	3 bread, 1 meat, 4 fat
French fries (small)	2 bread, 3 fat
Beef taco	1 bread, 1¼ meat, 1½ fat

Combination Foods

Casseroles (1 cup)	2 starch, 2 meat, 1 fat
Macaroni and cheese (1 cup)	2 starch, 1 meat, 2 fat
Spaghetti and meatballs (1 cup)	2 starch, 1 meat, 1 fat
Beans, peas, lentils (1 cup)	2 starch, 1 meat
Chili with beans (1 cup)	2 starch, 1 meat, 2 fat
Chow mein (2 cups)	1 starch, 2 vegetables, 2 meat
Cheese pizza (¼ of 10″)	2 starch, 1 meat, 1 fat
Bean soup (1 cup)	1 starch, 1 vegetable, 1 meat

Vegetable-type soups (10¾ oz.)	1 starch, 1 vegetable, 1 meat
Cream soups (1 cup)	1 starch, 1 fat
Sugar-free pudding (with skim milk)	1 starch
Coffee cake (med.)	2 bread, 3 fat
Chips (1 oz.)	1 starch, 1 fat

"Adapted with permission from *Exchange Lists for Weight Management* © 1989, American Diabetes Association, The American Dietetic Association."

RECORDING YOUR PROGRESS

You can design your menus and record what you actually eat on the same piece of paper. This will take less of your time by doing two steps in one. Initially, to insure that you are eating all of the daily food exchanges you are entitled to, no more no less, it is important to preplan what, where, and when you will eat. Use the Daily Food Diary to do just this. Make about fifty copies of this page to get you through the first few months of dieting. After regimenting yourself for this period of time, your diet will be second nature to you and preplanning will not be as essential.

To use this form, fill in the amount of calories you are trying to consume per day. Next, record the number of exchanges you may eat for this amount of calories as given in the chart on page 33. Now divide up those exchanges as desired and in a schedule that suits your lifestyle. Try to spread your food exchanges out over the whole day instead of eating just once or twice.

You are now ready to fill in the blanks for tomorrow's menu with selections from the food exchange lists. Have fun with this, and try to get the most taste for your exchanges. Plan your diet with confidence, knowing that it contains all necessary nutrients and will promote health and vitality.

Remember that a food diary is for your benefit. Nothing works here but honesty. Record both successful and less than successful days. Use this tool to reveal to yourself how much food goes into your mouth. It can often be surprising.

Now, here are a few sample menus you may use as an example for the 120 calorie menu. If you need greater or fewer calories than 1200, simply adjust exchanges according to the chart on page 33.

Daily Food Diary

Calories allowed per day _____
Exchanges allowed per day:

Starch _____ Meat _____ Dairy _____ Fruit _____ Fat _____
(Low-cal vegetables are free. Must eat
2 cups minimum per day)

Number of exchanges	Menu for Day _____	Exercise, Positive Changes

Breakfast
  starch _____
  meat _____
  milk _____
  fruit _____
  veg. _____
  fat _____		

Snack _____ _____		

Lunch
  starch _____
  meat _____
  milk _____
  fruit _____
  veg. _____
  fat _____		

Snack _____ _____		

Dinner
  starch _____
  meat _____
  milk _____
  fruit _____
  veg. _____
  fat _____		

Snack _____ _____		

1200 Calories (for weight loss)		1800 Calories (for weight maintenance)	
Number of exchanges	**Menu for Day** _3_	**Number of exchanges**	**Menu for Day** _3_
Breakfast starch _2_ meat _1_ milk ___ fruit _1_ veg. ___ fat _1_	1 English muffin 1 egg, cooked, no oil ½ cup orange juice hot tea 2 tsp. diet margarine	*Breakfast* starch _2_ meat _2_ milk ___ fruit _1_ veg. ___ fat _1_	1 English muffin 2 eggs, cooked, no oil ½ cup orange juice 2 tsp. diet margarine hot tea
Snack _____ _____		*Snack* ___2 fruits___ ___2 starch___	1 banana 3 whole graham crackers
Lunch starch _1_ meat _1_ milk _1_ fruit _1_ veg. _3_ fat _1_	Chef salad w/vegetables, cottage cheese, ham, low-cal dressing & croutons 1 cup fresh strawberries	*Lunch* starch _1_ meat _1_ milk _1_ fruit _2_ veg. _3_ fat _2_	Chef salad w/vegetables, cottage cheese, ham, low-cal dressing & croutons 1 roll 1 tsp. margarine 1 cup fruit salad
Snack ___2 fruit___ _____	1 large apple	*Snack* ___1 fruit___ _____	1 large apple
Dinner starch _1_ meat _3_ milk ___ fruit ___ veg. _2_ fat _1_	1 BBQ chicken breast, no skin ½ cup skinny french fries ½ cup green beans sliced tomatoes	*Dinner* starch _3_ meat _3_ milk ___ fruit ___ veg. _2_ fat _2_	1 BBQ chicken breast, no skin 1 cup skinny french fries* w/catsup green beans, sliced tomatoes ½ cup frozen yogurt
Snack ___1 starch___ ___1 milk___	1½ graham crackers 8 oz. ½% milk	*Snack* ___1 starch___ ___1 milk___	¾ cup All-Bran cereal 8 oz. ½% milk

*Indicates recipes included in this book.

1200 Calories (for weight loss)		1800 Calories (for weight maintenance)	
Number of exchanges	**Menu for Day** _5_	**Number of exchanges**	**Menu for Day** _5_

Breakfast
starch __1__
meat ____
milk __1__
fruit __1__
veg. ____
fat __1__
	1 bran or oat-bran
	   muffin; lowfat
	8 oz. ½% milk
	¼ cantaloupe
		Breakfast
		starch __2__
		meat ____
		milk __1__
		fruit __2__
		veg. ____
		fat __2__
			2 bran or oat-bran
			   muffins *
			8 oz. ½% milk
			½ cantaloupe

Snack _____ _____		*Snack* _____ _____	

Lunch
starch __2__
meat __2__
milk ____
fruit ____
veg. __1__
fat __1__
	Whopper, Jr., no mayo
	   (Burger King)
		Lunch
		starch __4__
		meat __3½__
		milk ____
		fruit ____
		veg. __1__
		fat __2__
			Whopper, no mayo
			   (Burger King)
			Side salad
			   with lowfat dressing

Snack __2 fruit__ _____	1 medium banana	*Snack* __2 fruit__ _____	1 medium apple

Dinner
starch __2__
meat __3__
milk ____
fruit __1__
veg. __2__
fat __1__
	3 oz. baked orange
	   roughy or other fish
	1 cup rice pilaf
	1 cup fresh green beans
	salad with lowfat dressing
	sugar-free gelatin with
	   fruit
		Dinner
		starch __2__
		meat __3__
		milk ____
		fruit __1__
		veg. __2__
		fat __2__
			4 oz. baked orange
			   roughy *
			1 cup rice pilaf *
			fresh green beans
			salad with lowfat
			   dressing
			gelatin salad with fruit

Snack __1 milk__ _____	8 oz. ½% milk	*Snack* __1 starch__ __1 milk__	1 serving favorite cereal 8 oz. ½% milk

*Indicates recipes included in this book.

1200 Calories (for weight loss)		1800 Calories (for weight maintenance)	
Number of exchanges	**Menu for Day 6**	**Number of exchanges**	**Menu for Day 6**
Breakfast starch _1_ meat ____ milk _1_ fruit _2_ veg. ____ fat ____	¾ cup high-fiber cereal 8 oz. ½% milk 1 whole banana	*Breakfast* starch _2_ meat ____ milk _1_ fruit _2_ veg. ____ fat _1_	¾ cup high-fiber cereal 8 oz. ½% milk 1 whole banana 1 pc. whole-wheat toast 2 tsp. diet margarine
Snack _____ _____		*Snack* _____ _____	
Lunch starch _2_ meat _1_ milk ____ fruit _1_ veg. _3_ fat _1_	large bowl clear vegetable-beef soup (some potatoes) salad, no-oil dressing whole-grain roll ½ cup fruit salad	*Lunch* starch _2_ meat _1_ milk ____ fruit _2_ veg. _3_ fat _1_	large bowl vegetable and beef soup (some potatoes) salad, lowfat dressing whole-grain roll 1 cup fruit salad
Snack _1 milk_ _____	8 oz. light, nonfat yogurt	*Snack* _1 milk_ _1 starch_	8 oz. light, nonfat yogurt 3 cups lowfat popcorn
Dinner starch _2_ meat _4_ milk ____ fruit ____ veg. _2_ fat _2_	4 oz. filet mignon large baked potato 1 Tbsp. light sour cream 2 tsp. diet margarine 2 Tbsp. grated cheese steamed broccoli salad with lowfat dressing	*Dinner* starch _3_ meat _4_ milk ____ fruit ____ veg. _2_ fat _4_	4 oz. filet mignon large baked potato 1 Tbsp. light sour cream 2 tsp. diet margarine 2 Tbsp. grated cheese 1 dinner roll steamed broccoli
Snack _1 fruit_ _____	½ cup grapes	*Snack* _1 starch_ _1 fruit_	2 pc. lite toast with apple butter

Develop New Eating Strategies

If you have always been one of those compulsive, do-it-by-the-book, perennial dieters, you will find that the eating program you are about to embark on has an appalling lack of structure. And right-fully so. Listen to what some other professionals are saying about dieting in an article from *Environmental Nutrition*. "We need to promote positive eating behavior without telling people [exactly] how much to eat," and "Breaking the diet-binge cycle is crucial before changes can be made in what people eat,"[4] so says Deborah Roussos R.D., M.D.

I could not agree more with Dr. Roussos. We are learning about a lifestyle that includes healthy eating patterns for life. In fact, there should be little difference between your normal daily diet and your weight-loss diet except for portion sizes. The types of foods you choose while losing weight should be the same foods incorporated into a maintenance program. You may certainly add a few extra frills along with the extra calories you will enjoy during maintenance, but a lowfat diet should be for keeps. The key is to have a willingness to learn and then act upon your newfound nutrition knowledge about what your body needs as fuel.

SUPERMARKET STRATEGIES

A substantial number of the food choices you make occur before you sit down to the table. Being a successful supermarket detective and developing the ability to decipher truth from fallacy must be one of your long-term goals.

Here's just one example. A well-known actress makes video advertisements for a whole wheat cracker as being healthful because it is baked instead of fried. Viewers want to believe this likable person; yet unless they know how to determine the percent of the calories coming from fat, they are at the mercy of the marketers who set this whole thing up. Packages and advertisements should not be your litmus test for whether or not a product is a healthy choice.

Here's another well-advertised example. Most peanut butters advertise that they contain "no cholesterol." What they don't tell you is that they are loaded with saturated fat that turns into cholesterol in your body. Or how about the turkey bologna we looked at in chapter 1? In actuality, that turkey bologna is only 25 percent fat-free—three-quarters of the product is pure fat!

How can they get away with this, you may ask? Simple. Labeling guidelines are not stringent enough and many manufacturers are absolute masters at distorting the truth.

Ultimately, you will find many wonderful, great-tasting foods that will serve you well both during weight loss and maintenance at your local supermarket. Remember, the foods you are learning to buy for weight loss should appear on your shopping list next year too.

TAMING THE PANTRY MONSTER

Beyond trickery, there is yet another major issue concerning your shopping cart. Picture this: you are alone in the house; that is, just you and the fridge (or the pantry will do). Everyone else is asleep or out for the evening. Or perhaps you live by yourself and you face this difficult dilemma every evening. Maybe you have had a tough day or have just been stood up by a friend. Or maybe it is a cold and blustery Friday night and you just want to "veg out" in front of the TV and forget your cares. But your definition of "veg out" does not involve carrots and celery sticks. Instead, it includes whatever foods are available as a soothing elixir to chase away today's trials.

Perhaps you have bought a box of light desserts and eat the whole box. Or maybe you think that you are immune from having all those family goodies in the house. Or, perhaps you have bought something unusual because it was on "special" at the store, a deal you just couldn't turn down. We can justify the purchase of almost anything when we think we are saving money.

JUST SAY NO—TO THE CUTE LITTLE GIRL SCOUTS SELLING COOKIES

I know, I know—this sounds cruel. The truth is, though, we give ourselves permission to eat all sorts of things because we are tricked into buying them for "a good cause." What about the special Easter-colored peanut M & M's that appear every March? Think about all the special events in our lives.

January—New Year's Day, Girl Scout cookies
February—Valentine's Day, chocolate hearts
March—Easter baskets and candies
April—More Easter specialties
May—Memorial Day barbecue
June—Summer vacation
July—Fourth of July picnic
August—More summer getaways
September—Labor Day weekend
October—Halloween candy
November—Thanksgiving foods and dinners
December—Christmas and other holiday celebrations, New
               Year's Eve

The list above does not even include birthdays, anniversaries, and all the other special events of your life. It's not that I want to stymie your fun; I am just saying that if we give ourselves permission to indulge with every "special occasion," we are constantly choosing to break our new healthy lifestyle.

Moral of the story: Don't think that you are punishing yourself or your family when Christmas chocolate kisses, Easter M & M's, and Girl Scout cookies do not appear in your pantry. After all, if the temptation isn't in the house when you get those 10:00 P.M. urges, your chances of surviving the pantry monster are much better.

Now let's look at some basic obstacle-course training for getting through your local supermarket unscathed.

BASIC GUIDELINES FOR GROCERY SHOPPING AND FOOD SELECTION

1. Don't ever go food shopping when you are hungry, tired, depressed, or craving something that is a very poor food choice. If this is simply not possible, you may have groceries delivered by many metropolitan supermarkets. Check for this service in your community by calling the manager's office of your local store.

2. Do not overbuy or overstock. Foods lose some of their nutritional value when stored too long, and you feel compelled to eat things so they will not "go to waste."

3. Resist the temptation to buy poor food choices merely because they are on special. Good food choices are also on special; choose them instead.

4. Don't buy junk food for the rest of the family. Nobody needs that stuff. Plus, you know and I know who will really eat a large portion of "the kids' cookies." Right?

5. Lite, light, and reduced-calorie alternatives are frequently just the right choice. They will allow you to have flavors you like without all the calories and fat. Analyze each food label for its own merit.

6. You can't go wrong with fresh fruits and vegetables. It is hard to overdo this group of foods. (You can overdo fruit juice which goes down quickly and is packed with sugar.) Avocados are the only fruit or vegetable with a substantial amount of fat. One-quarter of an

avocado contains ten grams of fat, or the amount found in about a tablespoon of butter.

THE FOOD GROUPS: CHOOSING MORE OF THE BEST AND LESS OF THE REST

You do not have to go to specialty stores or organic health food stores to shop nutritiously. Good nutrition is as close as the corner market. Do attempt to go to a place where the produce is always fresh and affordable. This will be a mainstay in your diet.

In this next section, you might want to make out your grocery shopping list. Foods are listed by food groups, and pros and cons of different choices are discussed.

BREADS, GRAINS, CEREALS, STARCHES

Breads, starches, cereals, and grains that contain only small amounts of sugar and fat are your best food selections overall. Foods in this category usually contain about 10 percent fat and can be seasoned well without fattening additives. Care should be taken, however, not to overdo a good thing. Do not exceed your daily recommended number of exchanges for this group (see pages 00 and 00). Only if you are involved in endurance sports should you eat more of these foods than are recommended.

- Almost all breads are very low in fat. Choose whole grain products that will add fiber and nutrients to your diet.
- Reduced-calorie breads allow you to have two slices for the calorie equivalent of only one slice. Many are also rich in fiber and make you feel full. Some companies offer hamburger buns that are light (eighty calories for the whole bun).
- High-fat breads include doughnuts, biscuits, croissants, sweet rolls, and other confectioneries including cookies and cakes.

- Cake, muffin, and bread mixes can contain fat even though they are a dry mix. Look for mixes advertising that they are lower in fat. Use angel food cake for a nice lowfat dessert.

- Making your own pasta, rice, and potato dishes from scratch will usually save you calories and fat. Many of the prepackaged mixes contain a lot more than starch; they contain hidden fat. Shells and Cheese by Velveeta contains 220 calories per one-half cup serving. Is this really what you want to put into your body? Try spaghetti with tomato sauce instead.

- Most cereals, with the exception of granola types, are very low in fat. They differ in calorie content greatly, however. A typical serving size can range from one-quarter cup (Grapenuts) to one-and-one-quarter cups (corn flakes). Cereal with skim milk or nonfat yogurt is a great way to start the day.

- Most granola type cereals contain 30 to 40 percent fat, which is above our 25 percent standard. But most of the flaked cereals are very low in fat, unless they contain nuts. Nuts are almost all fat. Check individual food labels for details.

- Starchy vegetables include potatoes, corn, rice, dried beans, peas, and some winter squashes. These are wonderfully healthy, but many people just eat too much of these. Another common mistake is to eat them smothered with butter, cheese, or another heavy source of fat.

- High-fiber foods from the bread and cereal group include whole grains, brown rice, bran cereals (wheat, oat, corn, rice bran, and others), and legumes (dried peas and beans). Inclusion of these items in your diet will help fill your stomach and satisfy your appetite.

- Good cracker choices include Melba rounds and toast, graham crackers, fat-free saltines, rice cakes, whole grain and lowfat crackers, and others that are less than 30 percent fat.

BREAD, GRAINS, CEREALS, AND STARCHES

Not Recommended	Recommended
Breads: commercial biscuits, muffins, sweet rolls, cornbread, French toast, and waffles are usually made with a lot of fat (make them at home instead, using lowfat recipes) *Cereals:* be careful about granola *Grains:* commercial rice mixes, potato mixes, macaroni and cheese mixes, and starter kits for skillet dinners (check the labels, some may be good choices) *Starchy foods* eaten out that contain large amounts of butter, cheese, or sour cream	*Breads:* whole wheat, white, rye, pumpernickel, oatmeal, raisin, Italian, whole grain breads; also English muffins, crumpets, matzo, egg or cheese bread (if it is a yeast product), pancakes; lower fat crackers (use your fat solutions equation on page 12) *All cereals:* watch fat content of granola; use sugary cereals sparingly or as a sweet snack *Grains:* white and brown rice and all other types of rice, all types of pasta (no high fat sauces), egg noodles, all types of flour; baked goods and other products made at home with less fat as compared with commercial varieties *Starchy vegetables:* including potatoes, corn, split peas, black-eyed peas, kidney beans, navy beans, black beans, lentils, garbanzos, lima beans, pinto beans, and all other types of dried peas and beans

MEAT, POULTRY, AND FISH

Choosing lowfat foods from this group can greatly enhance your chances of dieting success. Nothing could be more perfect for the dieter than, for example, a piece of grilled redfish with lemon and herbs. High-protein foods will help stabilize your blood glucose for a longer period of time and keep you from getting hungry.

I am not negative about vegetarianism, but consider that a bowl of rice and beans has more than 350 calories and contains less protein than the five-ounce piece of broiled fish containing only 200 calories. Also, if you are a vegetarian, keep in mind that you cannot make nonsensical choices such as a bag of cheese puffs instead of a tuna sandwich.

Though fish is the best choice, beef, pork, and poultry are also good under the circumstances described below.

- Fish is the lowest in calories and fat. Also, the protective omega-3 fatty acids are found in the fattier fish, including salmon, tuna, mackerel, sea trout, bluefish, herring, bonito, pompano, and anchovies.
- Beef is labeled and graded according to the fat content. "Select" is the leanest, followed by "choice." The leanest beef cuts include ground round, eye of the round steak or roast, and round steak. When a more tender cut is desired, both tenderloin and sirloin are still considered lean.
- Do not eat poultry skin. Also, do not cook a dish such as chicken and rice with the skin on, since the fat will be absorbed by the rice.
- Dark meat of chicken, skinned, has about the same amount of cholesterol as a very lean piece of beef. The lean beef still contains more saturated fat, however, than the poultry.
- When buying ground turkey, inquire whether or not ground turkey skin has been used in the preparation process. This can nullify all the good you are trying to accomplish.
- Shrimp, lobster, and sardines contain significantly higher amounts of fat and cholesterol than other types of fish, though there is controversy over whether this cholesterol is harmful to humans.
- Pork is different today than it once was. You can include Canadian bacon, pork chops, and boiled ham in a well-balanced and lowfat diet.
- New "lite" meats from younger animals have had less time to develop interstitial fat. They are a good lowfat choice as is veal.
- Choose healthy cooking methods, including broiling, grilling, baking, roasting, and boiling. Avoid frying.

- Eat beef if you want to. Remember that lean beef, pork, and lamb are not much higher in dietary cholesterol than is poultry.

- Avoid goose, duck, organ meats of all kinds, bacon, sausage, canned meats (except fish packed in water), hot dogs (beef, pork, and turkey—they are all fatty), bologna, salami, corned beef, pastrami, pickle loaf, and all other processed meats that are not made from fillets.

- Sandwich meats that are good lowfat choices include turkey breast, chicken breast, roast beef, Danish-style or boiled ham, and tuna. If you are trying to avoid the high sodium content of these foods, you may rinse a slice of smoked turkey (or other choice) under tap water, pat dry, and use as usual. This decreases the sodium content by half.

Meat Substitutes

- Meat substitutes may be used effectively for weight-loss and weight-control diets. If you do so, a vitamin/mineral supplement that includes iron, other trace minerals, and vitamin B-12 should be taken.

- All meats, dairy products, and eggs contain complete protein sources. That is, they contain all of the essential amino acids that humans cannot make themselves. Tofu (or soybean curd) is also a very good source of protein. Other protein foods such as legumes, vegetables, and nuts must be combined in such a way that they will provide the needed amino acids. If you are a serious vegetarian, you will need a book on this subject to help you with these combinations.

- One cup of cooked beans (pinto, black, navy, black-eyed, garbanzo, kidney) provides about the same amount of protein as three ounces of meat. An average cup of cooked beans contains about 200 calories while three ounces of lean chicken, fish, pork, or beef contains about 180 calories. I recommend using the lowest fat meats with an emphasis on fish as being more effective than either using beans or higher fat meats while losing weight.

- One egg contains five grams of fat and about 250 mg. of cholesterol. Eggs remain a good source of complete protein, however, and may stay in the diet of those who do not have a problem with elevated cholesterol levels.

- Peanut butter is about 85 percent fat and should be avoided. One serving contains only seven grams of protein, about the amount found in a quarter cup of cottage cheese. This is a very poor use of limited calories.

MEATS, POULTRY, FISH, AND SUBSTITUTES

Not Recommended	Recommended
Meats: regular ground beef, arm or chuck roast, ribs, fatty meats, heavily marbled meats, bacon, hot dogs (even turkey or all-beef franks), sausages, Vienna sausage, cold cuts if from chopped and pressed meats, corned beef and pastrami, all organ meats (heart, kidney, liver, sweet breads), commercially fried foods, meats canned or frozen with sauces or gravies (unless specified as lowfat) *Poultry:* goose, duck, poultry skin *Fish:* caviar and all fish roe *Meat Substitutes:* egg yolks (if you have a problem with cholesterol), peanut butter and other nut butters; pork and beans	*Meats:* lean beef (round steak, eye of the round roast, ground round), veal, luncheon meats, including turkey breast, chicken breast, roast beef, tuna, and lean ham *Poultry:* chicken (no skin), turkey *Fish:* all fish, clams, scallops, lobster, crab *Meat Substitutes:* "lite" meats, egg white, egg substitutes, tofu, soy-protein substitutes

FRUITS AND JUICES

Rediscover the freshness and appealing flavor of a great piece of fruit in its prime. The food diaries of many troubled dieters I have seen in my office reveal an elimination of fruit from their diet just because "they didn't think about it." Well, think about the fact that you can have two cups of fresh strawberries for about the same amount of calories as one chocolate chip cookie.

You may eat any fruit you like in the quantities specified on the exchange charts listed on page 33. Have fun at the grocery store knowing that you can buy anything you like.

- With the exception of avocados, fruits do not contain fat.
- Most fruits (except dried) are forty to sixty calories per one-half to one-cup serving.
- High levels of vitamin C can be found in tangerines, oranges, grapefruit, other citrus, avocados, strawberries, honeydew melon, guava, papaya, cantaloupe, mango, and kiwi fruit.
- High levels of vitamin A are found in apricots, cantaloupe, pink grapefruit, nectarines, persimmons, and papaya.
- Oranges, grapefruit, and bananas are very good sources of potassium.
- Certain fruits are high in fiber, including all berries, nectarines, pomegranates, apples, pears, figs, and prunes.
- Don't let fruits sit around. Eat them soon after purchase for the optimal nutritional value.
- Whole fruits are always better nutritional choices than are juices. They provide more fiber and usually more nutrients. And they also contribute toward that feeling of satiety to a greater extent.
- Fruit leathers and roll-ups can be a sugary treat that satisfies your sweet tooth. Some of the commercial varieties such as Betty Crocker® FRUIT ROLL-UPS®, which you might buy for your kids, can be a good choice for you too. Most contain about fifty calories per serving.
- Fruit products labeled "cocktails and drinks" are frequently nothing more than sugar water with a small amount of juice.

- Look for all-natural fruit spreads (on toast), such as Smucker's Simply Fruit® as an alternative to danish and sweet rolls.
- Retain skins on fruit when they are edible, but wash them thoroughly prior to eating.
- Don't overdo juice. It is more calorie concentrated than most sodas. On average, half a cup of juice (four ounces) has sixty calories.

FRUITS AND JUICES

Not Recommended	Recommended
Avoid dried fruits if you are sulfite sensitive. Don't drink too much juice. More than a few tablespoons of avocado or guacamole.	All fresh, canned, frozen, or dried fruit as well as juices may be used; avocado should be used in small amounts, never using more than one quarter of the fruit per meal; melons and strawberries are some of the least calorie-concentrated fruits.

VEGETABLES

This entire category of foods is a great way to fill your stomach without refilling those fat cells. All vegetables are recommended and are virtually fat-free. I think I have already said that every successful dieter I know has developed a healthy appetite for vegetables and incorporates something from this group at the noon and evening meal everyday. You get more nutrition for fewer calories in this group than with any other food. These are what you call high-nutrient density foods.

- Vegetables rich in vitamin A include carrots, sweet potatoes (consider this a starch), winter squash, tomatoes, and most dark leafy vegetables, including spinach, greens, and broccoli. Vitamin A is an antioxidant.

- Rich sources of vitamin C include tomatoes, brussels sprouts, cabbage, green peppers, and other varieties of peppers, kale, spinach, and greens. Vitamin C is an anti-oxidant.

- Folic acid is found in green leafy vegetables, asparagus, broccoli, and mushrooms.

- Consider the starchy vegetables as part of the bread group. Don't think of them as low-cal foods that you can load up on. Remember, corn, potatoes, and the other starchy vegetables are more like bread than they are like broccoli.

- Cruciferous vegetables, which are thought to help prevent certain gastrointestinal cancers, include brussels sprouts, broccoli, kohlrabi, cabbage, and cauliflower.

- Retain skins on vegetables whenever possible, but wash them thoroughly prior to eating.

- Use liberal amounts of fresh herbs, including parsley, cilantro, ginger, garlic, and onion to season foods tastefully without salt.

- Most of the light-colored vegetables, including iceberg lettuce, celery, and zucchini, have very few nutrients or fiber. Instead, use fresh spinach for salads to give your diet the nutrients it needs.

- To make salad preparation easier on evenings when you are too exhausted to wash the carrots, precut finger-food vegetables for dips and/or salads and store in airtight plastic bags and containers.

- Be careful of frozen vegetable mixes, which have a "sauce" or "seasoning packet." These may contain large sources of fat. Check your food label to make sure your choice is low in fat.

- *Eat at least four servings of food from this group every day!* There are virtually no maximum limits for this group of foods.

VEGETABLES

Not Recommended	Recommended
Buttered, creamed, or fried vegetables.	Any fresh, frozen, or canned vegetable without added fat may be eaten liberally. Especially low calorie and nutritious choices include spinach, greens, cabbage, broccoli, cauliflower, brussels sprouts, peppers, carrots, tomatoes, asparagus, and green beans.

SOUPS

Hot liquids help quench hunger pains. You can begin every meal with a bowl of soup made out of low-calorie vegetables if you like. (See page 39 for the vegetables list and page 230 for a recipe you can make yourself.) You are much better off having soups made at home, since you don't really know what has gone on in the kitchen of most restaurants.

- Choose all types of soup with a clear base. They can have noodles, vegetables, and meats and still be a better choice than a commercially prepared cream soup (especially when at a restaurant).

- If sodium intake is a concern, choose the new low-sodium varieties.

- Grocery store canned, creamed soup such as cream of mushroom, potato, chicken, or celery, are primarily thickened with flour and corn starch. These may be used by themselves or in recipes. When cooking them for soup, mix with skimmed milk.

- Avoid cheddar or cheese soup of any kind when eating out. When purchasing in a grocery store, check the label for fat content.

SOUPS

Not Recommended	Recommended
Cheese soups of all kinds, commercial cream soups, creamy clam chowder (unless made at home with accepted ingredients), commercially prepared beef stew or other soups with substantial amounts of beef in a thick gravy.	Bouillon, clear broth, lowfat vegetable soups, cream soups made from skimmed milk and thickened with starch, packaged dehydrated soups, minestrone, all soups made with a clear base and which do not appear to have substantial amounts of fat.

DAIRY PRODUCTS

Dairy products are another source of complete protein, as are meats, poultry, and fish. In fact, only animal products provide a complete protein in a single food.

Adults need calcium and phosphorous from dairy products as much as children do. Though whole milk is out of the question, a glass of skimmed milk is a dieter's bargain for only eighty calories. This milk can either be drunk fresh or made into pudding, gravy, or soup. Incorporation of calcium into your diet will especially help prevent osteoporosis (thinning of the bones) for women in later years.

- Choose skim, 1/2 percent or 1 percent lowfat milk. Lowfat buttermilk is also a good choice.
- Nonfat yogurt (plain or flavored) is a good choice. Some of the flavored varieties contain large amounts of sugar and should be eaten sparingly or during maintenance. "Lite" versions of nonfat yogurt, artificially sweetened, may be used frequently.
- Use lower fat versions of cottage cheese and sour cream.
- Some new lower fat and fat-free cheeses are good choices. In general, about 80 percent of the calories in all brick and natural cheeses come from fat, thus these cheeses should be used sparingly. Kraft Free™ processed cheese singles are delicious on sandwiches and in sal-

ads. It also melts well for grilled cheese sandwiches and other recipes. Alpine Lace™ has some lower fat and a fat-free cheddar that is good on salads but does not melt well.

- Cream cheese is about 90 percent fat, the light Philadelphia™ cream cheese is still about 65 percent fat. Look for the new nonfat Philadelphia™ cream cheese in your area. Ask your grocer to stock it.

- Try using a very sharp flavored cheese, such as feta or extra sharp cheddar, in much smaller quantities to achieve the flavors you are looking for with smaller amounts.

- Try using canned, evaporated skimmed milk in recipes calling for cream.

DAIRY PRODUCTS

Not Recommended	Recommended
Milk: whole milk and whole milk products, whole evaporated or sweetened condensed milk, cream, ice cream, sour cream, cream cheese, light cream cheese, non-dairy substitutes for either coffee creamers or sour cream *Cheese:* regular creamed cottage cheese	*Milk:* skimmed (nonfat) milk, ½ percent milk, nonfat dry milk powder, evaporated skimmed milk, lowfat buttermilk *Nonfat yogurt* *Cheeses:* fat-free cheese, lowfat cottage cheese, nonfat cream cheese, yogurt cheese

FATS, OILS, AND DRESSINGS

Don't refeed your fat cells by eating too many foods from this group. In fact, you don't ever have to use these foods. There is enough fat in the other foods you eat that if you avoided these altogether you would still have a diet containing 15 to 20 percent fat. Look for hidden sources of fat in combination foods, and check those food labels using your equation for percentage of calories from fat on page 12.

- Virtually all oils and other sources of pure fat are a minimum of one hundred calories per tablespoon. This includes butter, margarine, cooking oils, shortening, lard, and meat fat. Fat content of the diet should not exceed 25 percent of the total calorie intake.

- If you do not have a problem with cholesterol, you may use butter. It has no more calories than a regular tub or stick margarine.

- Use polyunsaturated oils, including corn, safflower, sunflower, and soybean if you have some sort of heart disease.

- Use monounsaturated oils, including rapeseed, canola, and olive oils to bring down the overall serum cholesterol without causing the good cholesterol, HDL (high density lipoprotein), to also decrease. This can help improve what is known as your cholesterol/HDL ratio, which is the best statistical predictor of heart disease.

- Use nonstick cooking sprays as a substitute for other oils in many recipes. They, too, are oils, but because of their packaging can be sprayed in a very thin film over most cooking surfaces.

- Tropical oils (coconut and palm oils) are extremely saturated as are animal fats, and they should be highly limited.

- Look for reduced-calorie or fat-free dressings, some of which have less than 10 calories per serving. Try not to exceed 25 calories per tablespoon for salad dressing.

- Lite or reduced calorie mayonnaise and Miracle Whip type salad dressings are better choices than their full-fat alternatives.

- Regular salad dressings are totally out, unless you have no other choice. One salad-bar scoop full of thousand island, ranch, blue cheese, Italian oil and vinegar, or green goddess can be the same amount of calories as a small hamburger (about three hundred).

- *Use as little as possible from this group of foods.* You cannot use too little of this group as an adult. Simply, if you eat fat, it turns into fat, especially if you are genetically predisposed to obesity. Every tablespoon of any kind of fat (mayo, oil, margarine, butter, cream, salad dressings) is one hundred calories you don't need. The less you eat from this group the less you refill those fat cells!

FATS, OILS, AND DRESSINGS

Not Recommended	Recommended
All fats should be limited as much as possible; butter, lard, tropical oils, including palm and coconut oil, salt pork, suet, bacon, and meat drippings are high in saturated fat; commercial gravies and cream sauces (make lowfat renditions at home)	*Oils:* vegetable oils including corn, safflower, sunflower, soybean, olive, canola, and all others *Dressings:* lighter mayonnaise and salad dressing products or those that are totally fat free *Fats:* butter, margarine, diet margarine in limited quantities; cooking sprays and butter substitutes

DESSERTS, FROZEN DESSERTS, COOKIES, AND CANDIES

"Having your diet and eating cake too" *is* possible—if the right choices are made. Look for light recipes like the one on page 000, or try a commercially made product such as the ones listed below.

- Angel food cake is almost fat-free.
- Frozen fruit bars, sorbets, fruit ice have no dietary fat.
- Lower fat ice milks or those using the fat substitute, Simplesse, are all good choices.
- Nonfat frozen yogurt is an excellent dessert choice. Some, which are sugar-free, are suitable for diabetics and helpful to calorie counters.
- Frozen chocolate and fudge bars averaging one hundred calories or less per bar taste great and actually provide some good nutritional value.

- Graham crackers, arrowroot, gingersnaps, and animal crackers make reasonable choices when you have a sweet tooth.
- Nonfat candy choices include most hard candies and jelly beans, as well as divinity (without nuts), marshmallows, marshmallow creme, and candy corn type items. Try to avoid candy bars, chocolates, and nougat type candy.

DESSERTS, FROZEN DESSERTS, COOKIES, AND CANDY

Not Recommended	Recommended
Frozen desserts: whole ice cream *Candies:* any type of commercial candy bar, chocolate, or nougat *Cakes and cookies:* commercial cakes, pies, icings; desserts made with large amounts of fat (check label or recipe), filled cookies	*Frozen desserts:* nonfat frozen yogurts, lowfat ice milk, fruit ices, gelatin desserts, fruit whips, meringues *Candies:* pure sugar candy, gum drops, jelly beans, hard candy, marshmallows, mints, jelly, jam, syrup, honey, and sugars all in limited quantity *Cakes and cookies:* angel food cake, gingersnaps, graham crackers, animal crackers, arrowroot crackers.

PACKAGED SNACKS AND MISCELLANEOUS FOODS

For some of us, the greatest threat to our diet lies in this area. You can count on the fact that most instant packaged foods are poor, high-fat choices. There are exceptions, of course. Be prepared to make the right choice by giving it forethought and knowing the facts.

- Use popcorn from air poppers or the microwave without much added fat. Use your fat solution equation (page 12) to determine the fat content.
- Spray air popped popcorn with buttery-flavored PAM or sprinkle with Molly McButter for a rich but lowfat taste.

- Chips of all sorts are high in fat, including corn chips, potato chips, bagel chips, and cheese chips. Lower fat renditions of these chips are not always lowfat. Use your fat solutions equation to determine the percent fat in various food products for yourself.
- If you bring home chips, candy, snack crackers, and pastries, they will be eaten. No one needs them.
- Nuts are out. They range from 75 percent fat (peanuts) to 95 percent fat (macadamia nuts). Do not use nuts as a source of protein. They are really just repositories for fat. Avoid them altogether except when used in small quantities in recipes.
- Sour pickles contain very few calories and no fat. Although pickled foods are not recommended by the American Cancer Society because they may be slightly carcinogenic, they may be eaten occasionally.
- Olives are about 80 percent fat. Use them as a condiment instead of a munching food.

PACKAGED SNACKS AND MISCELLANEOUS FOODS

Not Recommended	Recommended
Most chips, even bagel chips, high-fat snack items appearing in vending machines.	Pretzels, lowfat popcorn, dried fruits and raisins, lowfat yogurts, fresh fruit, grapes, rice cakes, lower fat chip alternatives.

BEVERAGES

During the diet phase, there isn't much room for too many frills in this area. I usually recommend that all beverages besides milk be calorie-free so that you can achieve a diet that is high in nutrient density while low in calories.

There is no room in a diet program for alcoholic beverages. They are absolutely empty calories and can even drain your body of needed B-vitamins. Keep in mind also that if breast cancer runs in your family, even a few social, alcoholic cocktails per week can increase your chances of getting breast cancer.

I do cook with wine in some recipes. Since alcohol has a lower boiling point than water, the alcohol vaporizes quickly so that there is no alcohol left in the final recipe. It can act as a good flavor enhancer and meat tenderizer in beef and chicken recipes.

- Fruit smoothies are a great summertime treat. Make enough for the entire family (see page 223 for recipe).
- Become accustomed to sugar-free sodas. My favorites include diet Coke, sugar-free A & W root beer, and diet Shasta orange. Regular sugary sodas are out of the question if they are drunk on a regular basis.
- Avoid alcoholic beverages altogether while actively dieting. You may include one per day during weight maintenance, if necessary. Wine and light beer are better choices than a mixed cocktail or frozen drink.
- Water with a squeeze of lime or lemon is your best restaurant or at-home beverage.
- Drink eight 8-ounce glasses of a water-based beverage per day.
- Herbal teas make wonderful hot or cold beverages.
- If you prefer regular tea (try Constant Comment), dilute with extra water for less caffeine intake.

BEVERAGES

Not Recommended	Recommended
Sugary sodas, excessive sources of caffeine or artificial sweeteners, artificially colored and flavored drinks, Cremora, Coffeemate, other non-dairy creamers, alcoholic beverages	Coffee, tea, herbal teas, decaffeinated products, sugar-free carbonated beverages, fruit and vegetable juices, club soda, mineral water, plain seltzer, lemon water, nonfat evaporated dry milk for coffee creamer

LET'S GET SPECIFIC

In this section, I will give you some specific brand names of foods that are better choices given the criteria we have established. Keep in mind that this list will not be current forever, since new food products come and go. Ultimately, you can only depend on learning how to make these determinations for yourself.

Food	Size	Calories	Grams of Fat	% of Fat
Snacks				
Quaker Butter Popped Corn Cakes	3	105	0	0
Wege Honey Whole Wheat Pretzels with Sesame Seeds	1 oz.	110	.9	7
Pretzels	1 oz.	110	1	8
Roasted chestnuts	1 oz.	70	.6	8
Popcorn, plain air-popped	4 cups	100	1	9
American Grains Tortilla Bites	1 oz.	100	1	9
Guiltless Gourmet No Oil Tortilla Chips	1 oz.	110	1	11
Barbara's 9-Grain Pretzels	1 oz.	120	2	15
Crackle Rice Thins, French onion	6	36	1	25
Doritos Gourmet Chips, Light Cool Ranch flavor	1 oz.	130	4	28
New York Style Toasted Garlic Pita Chips	1 oz.	135	4	28
New York Style Bagel Chips	1 oz.	120	4	30
Pepperidge Farm Pretzel Goldfish	1 oz.	120	4	30
Ralston Chex Mix, cheddar cheese	1 oz.	130	5	35
Barbara's Pinta Chips	1 oz.	138	6	39
Popcorn, with oil and salt	4 cups	160	8	45
Tortilla chips, standard	1 oz.	155	8	46
Potato chips, standard	1 oz.	160	10	56
Cakes and Cookies				
Entenmann's Fat-Free, Cholesterol-Free banana crunch cake	1 oz.	80	0	0
Entenmann's Fat-Free, Cholesterol-Free cherry cheese pastry	1.3 oz.	90	0	0

Food	Size	Calories	Grams of Fat	% of Fat
Entenmann's Fat-Free, Cholesterol-Free chocolate loaf cake	1 oz.	70	0	0
Health Valley Fat-Free Apricot Delight Cookies	3	75	.3	4
Health Valley Fat-Free Raspberry Jumbos	1	70	.3	4
Nabisco Devil's Food Cakes	1	70	1	12
Nabisco Old-Fashioned Ginger Snaps	2	60	1	15
Nabisco Fig Newtons	2	120	2	15
Nabisco Honey-Maid Cinnamon Grahams	4	120	2	15
FFV Devil's Food Trolley Cakes	2	120	2	15
Sunshine Animal Crackers	13	120	3	22
Nabisco Chocolate Chip Snaps	3	70	2	25
Nabisco Famous Chocolate Wafers	2.5	70	2	25
FFV Whole Wheat Fig Fruit Bars	1	70	2	26
Health Valley Ranch Fruit Chunks Raisin Oat Bran	2	70	2	26
Nabisco Strawberry Newtons	1	70	2	26
Estee Oatmeal Raisin	4	120	4	30
Nabisco Honey-Maid Graham Bites Apple Cinnamon	4	120	4	30
Nabisco Nilla Wafers	7	120	4	30
Nabisco Teddy Grahams	11	60	2	30
Nabisco My Goodness Banana Nut Cookies	1	90	3	30
Barnum's Animal Crackers	5	60	2	30
Nabisco Almost Home Oatmeal Raisin	1	70	3	38
Nabisco Biscos Sugar Wafers	4	70	3	38

Frozen Desserts

Food	Size	Calories	Grams of Fat	% of Fat
Sealtest Free, chocolate, strawberry vanilla	1 cup	200	0	0
Sealtest Free dessert bar, chocolate with fudge swirl	2.5 oz.	90	0	0
Sealtest Free dessert bar, vanilla with fudge swirl	2.5 oz.	80	0	0
Centrone's Italian Ice	1 cup	185	0	0
Lucerne Fat-Free Frozen Dairy Dessert Chocolate Crunch Royale	1 cup	200	0	0
Dole Fruit 'N' Juice Bar, Strawberry	1	70	trace	trace

Food	Size	Calories	Grams of Fat	% of Fat
Dole Fruit 'N' Yogurt Bar, Strawberry-Banana	1	60	trace	trace
Simple Pleasures, chocolate	1 cup	280	1	3
Simple Pleasures, strawberry, coffee	4 oz.	120	.5	3
Dole Sorbet, Strawberry	1 cup	200	1	4
Breyer's Lowfat Frozen Yogurt, Chocolate	1 cup	240	2	7
Weight Watcher's Chocolate Treat Bar	1	100	1	9
Edy's American Dream, Chocolate	1 cup	240	3	11
Weight Watcher's Vanilla Sandwich	1	150	3	18
Yoplait Soft Frozen Yogurt	1 cup	240	5	18

Crackers

Food	Size	Calories	Grams of Fat	% of Fat
Chico-San Rice Cakes	1	35	0	0
Ralston Purina, Rykrisp Bread, Natural Snack Crackers	2 triple	40	0	0
Wasa Crispbread, Hearty Rye	1	45	0	0
Ideal Crispbread Extra Thins	3	48	0	0
Nabisco Comet (Ice Cream) Cups	1	18	0	0
Finn Crisp, Dark	2	38	0	0
Kavli Norwegian Crispbread, thick	1.5	52	0	0
Manischewitz Unsalted Matzos	½	55	.2	3
Old London Onion Rounds	5	52	.17	3
Ryvita Crisp Bread, High Fiber	2	46	.2	4
Old London Unsalted White Melba Toast	3	51	.2	4
Carr's Whole Wheat Crackers	4	140	2	13
Sunshine Krispy Saltine Crackers	5	60	1	15
Sunshine Krispy Whole Wheat Saltine	5	60	1	15
Sunshine Oyster and Soup Crackers	16	60	1	15
JJ Flats, onion	1 oz.	120	2	15
Nabisco Oysterettes	18	60	1	15
Old London Whole Grain Rounds	5	54	1	17
Ralston Purina Rykrisp Brand Seasoned Crackers	2 triple	45	1	20
Crackle Bread	2	35	1	20
Nabisco Crown Pilot	1	70	2	25
Wasa Crispbread Fiber Plus	1	35	1	26
Burry Milk Lunch Crackers	2	70	2	26
Kavli Ultrathin Crispbread	3	33	1	27

Food	Size	Calories	Grams of Fat	% of Fat
Bremner Biscuit Whole Wheat Wafers	6	63	2	29
Nabisco Royal Lunch	1	60	2	30
Nabisco Premium Crackers, Unsalted Tops	5	60	2	30
Nabisco Triscuit Wafers	3	60	2	30
Pepperidge Farm Cheddar Cheese Goldfish	27	60	2	30
Nabisco Wheat Thins	8	70	3	38

Breads

Food	Size	Calories	Grams of Fat	% of Fat
Sara Lee Plain Bagel	1	230	1	4
Sara Lee Cinnamon and Raisin Bagel	1	240	2	8
Pillsbury Crusty French Loaf	1" slice	60	less than 1	less than 15
Pillsbury Soft Breadsticks	1	100	2	18
Pepperidge Farm Banana Nut Muffin	1	250	5	18
Pillsbury White Pipin' Hot Loaf	1" slice	80	2	23
Sara Lee Hearty Fruit Apple Oat Bran Muffin	1	190	6	28
Pepperidge Farm Cinnamon Swirl Muffin	1	190	6	28

Cereals

Food	Size	Calories	Grams of Fat	% of Fat
Frosted Mini-Wheats	1 oz.	110	0	0
Nutri-Grain Wheat	1 oz.	110	0	0
Grape Nuts	1 oz.	110	0	0
Post Natural Bran Flakes	1 oz.	90	0	0
Wheat Chex	1 oz.	100	0	0
Kellogg's Bran Flakes	1 oz.	90	0	0
Crispix	1 oz.	110	0	0
Kellogg's Corn Flakes	1 oz.	110	0	0
Fruitful Bran	1 oz.	90	0	0
Product 19	1 oz.	110	0	0
Rice Chex	1 oz.	110	0	0
Rice Krispies	1 oz.	110	0	0
Honey Smacks	1 oz.	110	0	0
Post Natural Raisin Bran	1 oz.	90	0	0
Apple Jacks	1 oz.	110	0	0
Frosted Flakes	1 oz.	110	0	0
Honey Nut Cheerios	1 oz.	110	1	8
Nabisco Shredded Wheat 'N' Bran	1 oz.	110	1	8

Food	Size	Calories	Grams of Fat	% of Fat

Salad Dressings

Food	Size	Calories	Grams of Fat	% of Fat
Kraft Free, Ranch	1 Tbsp.	16	0	0
Kraft Free, Thousand Island	1 Tbsp.	20	0	0
Kraft Free, Italian	1 Tbsp.	6	0	0
Kraft Oil-Free Italian	1 Tbsp.	4	0	0
Hidden Valley "Take Heart," Italian	1 Tbsp.	14	0	0
Hidden Valley "Take Heart," Thousand Island	1 Tbsp.	25	0	0
Wishbone "Lite" Italian	1 Tbsp.	6	0	0
Good Seasons (prepared from packet) Lite Zesty Italian	1 Tbsp.	25	2.5	9
Hidden Valley "Take Heart," Original Ranch	1 Tbsp.	20	1	45
Wishbone "Lite" Ranch	1 Tbsp.	45	4	80

Meats and Fish

Food	Size	Calories	Grams of Fat	% of Fat
Halibut, cod, cooked	3 oz.	120	1	8
Louis Rich, Turkey Breast	1 slice	23	.3	11
Louis Rich, Turkey Ham	1 slice	35	.4	12
Oscar Mayer, Corned Beef	1 slice	16	.3	16
Turkey, light meat, cooked, no skin	3 oz.	151	3	18
Shrimp, steamed, shelled	3 oz.	100	2	18
Chicken, light meat, cooked, no skin	3 oz.	142	4	25
Beef, round, lean, broiled	3.5 oz.	191	6.2	29
Louis Rich, Turkey Pastrami	1 oz.	33	1.2	32
Ham, sliced, lean (5% fat)	1 slice	37	1.4	34
Lamb, leg, lean, roasted	3 oz.	158	6	34
Turkey, 93% lean ground (cooked)	3 oz.	143	6	39

Milk

Food	Size	Calories	Grams of Fat	% of Fat
Milk, skim	8 oz.	90	1	10
Yogurt, nonfat, plain	½ cup	90	2	10
Milk, 1% lowfat	8 oz.	105	2	17
Cottage Cheese, lowfat	½ cup	90	2	20
Milk, 2% lowfat	8 oz.	120	5	37
Milk, 4% or whole	8 oz.	160	9	50

Cheese

Food	Size	Calories	Grams of Fat	% of Fat
Alpine Lace Free 'n' Lean (cheddar, mozzarella, American)	1 oz.	35	0	0
Kraft Free Singles	1 oz.	45	0	0

Food	Size	Calories	Grams of Fat	% of Fat
Polly-O Free, mozzarella	1 oz.	40	0	0
Polly-O Free, ricotta	1 oz.	25	0	0
Weight Watchers, Low Sodium	1 oz.	50	2	36
Tasty-Lo Pasteurized Process (onion or garlic)	1 oz.	50	2	36
Kaukauna Lite 50 cheese spread	1 oz.	70	3	38
Kraft, Light singles, Swiss	1 oz.	70	3	38
Kraft Light 'n' Lively, American Flavored	1 oz.	70	4	51
Borden's Lite-Line	1 oz.	52	3	52
Kraft Light Naturals, Mild, Reduced Fat	1 oz.	80	5	56
Mozzarella, part-skimmed milk	1 oz.	90	6	60

Fast Food

Food	Size	Calories	Grams of Fat	% of Fat
Arby's Roasted Chicken Breast	1	254	7	25
Arby's Hot Ham and Cheese	1	353	13	33
Arby's Roast Beef, Jr.	1	218	8	33
Burger King, BK Broiler without sauce	1	289	8	24
Chick-Fil-a, Chargrilled Chicken Deluxe Sandwich	1	266	5	16
Hardee's Grilled Chicken Sandwich	1	310	9	26
Jack-in-the-Box, Chicken Fajita Pita	1	292	8	25
Jack-in-the-Box, Club Pita	1	284	8	25
Kentucky Fried Chicken, Baked Beans	1	109	1	9
Kentucky Fried Chicken, Corn on the Cob	1	176	3	15
Kentucky Fried Chicken, Mashed Potatoes and Gravy	1	62	1	15
Long John Silver, Ocean Chef Salad	1	229	8	31
McDonald's Apple Bran Muffin	1	190	0	0
McDonald's Chocolate Lowfat Milk Shake	1	320	1.7	4
McDonald's Vanilla Frozen Yogurt Cone	1	100	.75	6
McDonald's Hamburger	1	260	10	35
Pizza Hut, Standard Cheese	2 med. slices	340	11	29
Pizza Hut, Superstyle Cheese	2 med. slices	410	14	31

Food	Size	Calories	Grams of Fat	% of Fat
Taco Bell, Pintos 'N' Cheese	1	168	5	27
Taco Bell, Bellbeefer	1	221	7	29
Taco Bell, Bean Burrito	1	343	12	31
Taco Bell, Combination Burrito	1	404	16	36
Taco Bell, Bellbeefer with cheese	1	278	12	39
Wendy's Baked Potato, plain	1	250	2	7
Wendy's, Chili	8 oz.	260	8	28
Wendy's, Small Hamburger	1	260	9	31
Wendy's, Grilled Chicken Sandwich	1	350	13	33

Instead of That . . .
Try This!

I have always believed that when something is taken away an alternative must be put in its place. This chapter is about tangible, edible alternatives. It is my goal that, at the end of this chapter, you can see that there are few foods which don't have some sort of lowfat substitute. We will talk about home-cooked meals, ingredients, fast foods, restaurant foods, and trigger foods. When you have studied the actual figures and recipes, you will see for yourself that you can enjoy most of your favorite foods and still lose weight.

I encourage you to check out the recipes in other books as well. There are many wonderful lowfat and low-calorie cookbooks, not to mention the 150 recipes in the first *Love Hunger* book. Develop a card system that allows you to save your favorite ones. There are really so many good recipes that it is easy to forget which you preferred.

WHAT TO WATCH FOR IN THESE SUBSTITUTES

As you go through the list, you will readily identify the roots of the typical high-calorie and extremely high-fat American diet. You will be amazed to see where fats come from in many of the foods that you once held dear. You will find that most of these meals exceed twelve hundred calories for a single meal and often contain more than 40 percent of the total calories as fat. In contrast, the alternatives never exceed 30 percent of the calories as fat and are lower in total calories. Though it is more difficult to control calorie and fat intake when eating out, many of the suggested meals in this chapter are at or under the 25-percent-fat mark. Remember, no matter what you eat, weight loss and weight maintenance will be easier when consuming no more than 25 percent of your total calories as fat.

Now let me really put this in perspective. Imagine that you have just sat down to a fine dinner. The china is out, soft music is playing in the background, and in the middle of your plate is a whole stick of butter, ringed in fresh parsley. In fact, this is your entrée for the night. You have some nice vegetables on the side, a potato, and a protein source as well. But at the center of it all is this stick of butter. You pick up your fork and knife and slice a pat of butter off the end of the hardened stick. You put it in your mouth and realize that there are yet twenty-three more bites ahead of you just like that one. How does it make you feel to think about eating twenty-four teaspoons of butter for dinner? In fact, many of the traditional restaurant meals have so much fat that it is equivalent to eating almost an entire stick of butter. The average stick of butter has ninety-seven grams of fat, and several of the meals shown in this chapter contain grams of fat in the high eighties and higher. It is no wonder we feel sick after a heavy meal with this kind of food going into our bodies.

Have an open mind as you go through this chapter. Recognize that the old ways are not an option. Changes must be made. Fried foods must be given up and replaced with good healthy choices. For your favorite high-fat foods, imagine all the butter you are *not* consuming. Finally, choose alternatives that you can learn to actually prefer over the old choices.

TRY THIS IN RESTAURANTS

STEAKHOUSE

Instead of That . . .			Try This!		
	Calories	Fat		Calories	Fat
8-ounce ribeye steak	825	47.1	4-ounce filet mignon,		
1 large baked potato	160	.2	no bacon	290	16.0
2 Tbsp. whipped butter	120	13.3	1 large baked potato	160	.2
1 Tbsp. sour cream	35	3.0	1 tsp. butter substitute		
2 Tbsp. grated cheddar			sprinkles*	10	.1
cheese	90	8.0	1 Tbsp. sour cream	35	3.0
Dinner salad	25	0	Dinner salad	25	0
2 Tbsp. Ranch dressing	160	11.6	1 ounce of diet salad		
1 wheat roll	100	2.0	dressing*	30	.1
1 tsp. margarine	35	3.7	Iced tea with lemon	0	0
4 ounces of red wine	100	0			
Total Calories	1650	88.9*	Total Calories	560	19.4
Approx. % calories			Approx. % calories		
from fat	47%		from fat	32%	

*Having 87 grams of fat or 756 calories of fat is like eating almost a whole stick of butter!

*Pack these items in your purse or pocket.

SEAFOOD

Instead of That . . .			Try This!		
	Calories	Fat		Calories	Fat
7 ounces batter-fried fish	700	25.0	6 ounces baked or		
3 Tbsp. tartar sauce	300	24.3	broiled fish with		
4 hush puppies	240	16.0	lemon	300	4.0*
½ cup coleslaw	130	7.3	½ cup green beans	30	1.0
French fries, large	290	19.0	½ cup rice pilaf	120	2.0
12-ounce soft drink	150	0	Whole wheat roll	100	2.0
			Coffee, iced tea	0	0
Total Calories	1810	91.6	Total Calories	550	9.0
Approx. % calories			Approx. % calories		
from fat	46%		from fat	16%	

*This meal contains the same amount of fat as a stick of butter!

*This number can range from 1 to 6 grams depending on the variety of fish.

ITALIAN PIZZA

Instead of That . . .	Calories	Fat	Try This!	Calories	Fat
4 pieces medium pizza, pepperoni, double cheese, thick crust	920	50.8	2 pieces medium cheese pizza with vegetable toppings, no olives	380	11.4
2 Tbsp. Parmesan cheese	46	3.0	Large side salad	35	0
Tea	0	0	3 Tbsp. fat-free Italian dressing	12	.2
			Tea	0	0
			1 peppermint	20	0
Total Calories	968	53.8	Total Calories	447	11.6
Approx. % calories from fat	50%		Approx. % calories from fat	23%	

BURGERS AND MORE

Instead of That . . .	Calories	Fat	Try This!	Calories	Fat
Quarter pound cheeseburger, typical	525	31.4	Grilled chicken sandwich with mustard, veggies, no mayo	320	8.9
French fries, large	353	19.0	Large salad	50	0
20-ounce soft drink	250	0	3 Tbsp. Reduced-calorie dressing	12	.2
Frozen dessert cone	200	5.6	Iced tea or diet soda	0	0
Total Calories	1328	56.0	Total Calories	382	9.1
Approx. % calories from fat	38%		Approx. % calories from fat	21%	

*This menu would have 47% of the calories from fat without the drink.

GREEK RESTAURANT

Instead of That . . .			Try This!		
	Calories	Fat		Calories	Fat
Moussaka, 4″ x 4″ x 2″	500	17.8	2 large or 4 small		
Greek salad, 1 oz. feta			dolmades with sauce	300	9.0
cheese, 2 greek			Vegetables of the day	100	2.0
olives, 2 Tbsp.			Greek salad, 1 oz. feta		
house dressing	257	25.2	cheese, 1 greek		
2 slices Greek bread	200	2.7	olive	80	6.5
1 Tbsp. Butter	108	12.2	1 slice Greek bread	100	1.3
Vegetables of the day	100	2.1	2 Tbsp. reduced-calorie		
Baklava, 1″ x 2″ x 1″	300	20.0	dressing	8	.1
			Iced tea with lemon	0	0
Total Calories	1465	80.0	Total Calories	588	18.9
Approx. % calories			Approx. % calories		
from fat	50%		from fat	30%	

CHINESE FOOD

Instead of That . . .			Try This!		
	Calories	Fat		Calories	Fat
6 ounces Sweet and			1 cup Moo Goo Gai Pan	255	8.0
Sour pork	450	25.0	1 cup steamed rice	223	.2
1 egg roll	280	5.0	1 cup hot and sour soup	75	0
Fried rice	230	5.0	1 fortune cookie	30	0
1 cup hot and sour soup	75	0	Hot tea with artificial		
1 fortune cookie	30	0	sweetener	0	0
Hot tea with 2 tsp. sugar	30	0			
Total Calories	1095	35.0	Total Calories	583	8.2
Approx. % calories			Approx. % calories		
from fat	31%		from fat	13%	

MEXICAN RESTAURANT

Instead of That . . .	Calories	Fat	Try This!	Calories	Fat
2 cheese enchiladas with chili	792	41.8	Chicken fajita salad (lettuce, tomato,		
3/4 cup Mexican Rice	160	3.2	shredded carrot,		
1/2 cup Refried Beans	135	1.4	onion, pico de gallo,		
20 tortilla chips, restaurant style	370	20.0	3 oz. meat, 1 oz. grated cheese,		
1/2 cup Picante sauce	30	0	picante sauce, no		
1 flour tortilla	150	3.0	other dressing)	271	10.1
1 tsp. butter	35	4.0	2 six-inch corn tortillas	134	2.2
Tea	0	0	Tea	0	0
Total Calories	1672	73.4	Total Calories	405	12.3
Approx. % calories from fat	40%		Approx. % calories from fat	27%	

BARBECUE

Instead of That . . .	Calories	Fat	Try This!	Calories	Fat
Barbecue brisket, 3 oz.	250	9.5	Barbecue breast of chicken, 4 oz., no		
2 oz. Barbecue sauce	200	15.5	skin	175	4.7
3/4 cup Beans	225	4.0	1/4 cup Barbecue sauce	48	.2
1/2 cup Potato salad	160	8.6	Corn on the cob	120	1.0
1 slice bread	80	1.0	1/2 cup coleslaw made		
1/4 cup Barbecue sauce	48	.2	with vinaigrette	30	.1
Tea	0	0	Iced tea	0	0
Total Calories	963	38.8	Total Calories	373	6.0
Approx. % calories from fat	36%		Approx. % calories from fat	14%	

ITALIAN

Instead of That . . .	Calories	Fat	Try This!	Calories	Fat
1½ cups lasagna	430	25.0	1½ cup spaghetti with tomato and meat sauce	337	13.0
2 slices garlic bread	216	6.3			
Dinner salad	25	0	Dinner salad	25	0
2 Tbsp. Italian dressing	168	14.7	2 Tbsp. low-calorie Italian dressing	8	.1
1 slice (3 oz.) carrot cake	326	17.1	1 slice Italian bread, no butter	90	1.0
Total Calories	1165	63.1	Total Calories	460	14.1
Approx. % calories from fat	49%		Approx. % calories from fat	28%	

SOUTHERN FARE

Instead of That . . .	Calories	Fat	Try This!	Calories	Fat
Chicken fried steak	580	37.0	3 oz. Beef pot roast with 1½ cups vegetables	250	6.0
¾ cup Mashed potatoes	167	6.6			
½ cup Cream gravy	70	4.6	¾ cup Green beans, with slight butter	46	2.0
¾ cup Green beans, butter seasoning	36	2.0	1 medium Sliced tomato	25	0
1 hot roll	85	2.1	1 roll, whole wheat	100	1.0
1 tsp. butter	36	4.1			
Cherry pie, ⅙ pie	282	11.7			
Tea, with sugar	40	0			
Total Calories	1296	68.1	Total Calories	421	9.0
Approx. % calories from fat	47%		Approx. % calories from fat	19%	

MORE SOUTHERN FARE

Instead of That . . .	Calories	Fat	Try This!	Calories	Fat
Fried chicken, 3 med. pieces	600	35.3	Roasted chicken, w/o skin, 6 oz.	296	7.7
½ cup Fried okra	190	8.7	½ cup Crookneck squash, ½ tsp. butter	33	2.0
¾ cup Scalloped potatoes	210	7.5	Brussels sprouts, ½ cup, butter ½ tsp.	60	2.0
Cornbread, 2" x 2" x 1"	130	3.0	1 slice Low-calorie bread, toasted	40	.5
1 tsp. butter	36	4.1	½ tsp. low-calorie margarine	8	1.0
½ cup Butter-pecan premium ice cream	310	24.0	½ cup ice milk	120	3.0
Coffee, ½ oz. creamer, and sugar	37	1.6	Coffee	0	0
Total Calories	1513	84.2	Total Calories	557	16.2
Approx. % calories from fat	50%		Approx. % calories from fat	26%	

COUNTRY BREAKFAST

Instead of That . . .	Calories	Fat	Try This!	Calories	Fat
Eggs, 2, scrambled with milk and butter	190	14.2	Eggs (½ cup Egg Beaters), scrambled in 1 tsp. low-cal margarine	67	2.0
Sausage, 2 patties	300	25.0	1 oz. lean Ham	80	2.7
½ cup hash browns	170	9.0	Sliced tomatoes	25	0
2 medium biscuits	220	9.0	2 slices low-calorie bread, toasted	80	1.0
2 tsp. butter	72	8.2	1 Tbsp. jam, sugar-free	25	0
1 Tbsp. jelly or jam	55	0	Coffee	0	0
Coffee with sugar and creamer	37	1.6			
Total Calories	1044	67.0	Total Calories	277	5.7
Approx. % calories from fat	58%		Approx. % calories from fat	18%	

SALAD BAR

Instead of That . . .	Calories	Fat	Try This!	Calories	Fat
Chef salad			Chef salad		
Lettuce, fresh			Lettuce, fresh		
spinach, other salad			spinach, other salad		
greens	30	0	greens	30	0
½ avocado	275	27.0	½ medium tomato	20	0
½ medium tomato	20	0	½ cup cucumber slices	7	0
2 oz. Danish ham	116	7.4	½ cup carrots, grated	35	0
2 oz. cheddar cheese	228	18.8	½ cup lowfat cottage		
6 sliced black olives	60	5.3	cheese	82	1.2
⅓ cup croutons	60	3.0	½ cup croutons	60	3.0
5 Tbsp. regular dressing	400	43.1	5 Tbsp. fat-free dressing	20	.4
1 bread stick, hot, baked	100	7.0	2 rye wafers	45	.2
1 cup cheddar and			1 cup beef/vegetable		
broccoli soup	272	21.5	soup	102	1.9
	———	———		———	———
Total Calories	1561	133.1	Total Calories	401	6.7
Approx. % calories			Approx. % calories		
from fat	77%		from fat	15%	

TRY THIS IN FAST FOOD RESTAURANTS

BURGER KING

Instead of That . . .			Try This!		
	Calories	Fat		Calories	Fat
Whopper, double beef			Whopper Jr., no mayo,		
with cheese	950	60.0	no cheese*	275	12.0
Regular French fries	227	13.0	Salad with low-cal		
Medium chocolate shake	320	12.0	dressing	38	.1
			20 oz. Diet cola	0	0
Total Calories	1497	85.0	Total Calories	313	12.1
Approx. % calories			Approx. % calories		
from fat	51%		from fat	35%	

*Mustard, catsup, pickles, lettuce, tomato and onion may always be used on hamburgers without significantly adding to the calorie content of the meal.

BURGER KING BREAKFAST

Instead of That . . .			Try This!		
	Calories	Fat		Calories	Fat
Scrambled Egg Platter			Croissandwich with ham		
with sausage	702	52.0	and egg, no cheese	265	14.0
Coffee with sugar and			Coffee	0	0
cream	37	1.6			
Total Calories	739	53.6	Total Calories	265	14.0
Approx. % calories			Approx. % calories		
from fat	65%		from fat	48%	

*This is still a high-fat item even though low in calories. There are not many fast food breakfast items that are low in fat. Some hotels and breakfast restaurants now serve egg substitute breakfasts.

JACK-IN-THE-BOX

Instead of That . . .			Try This!		
	Calories	Fat		Calories	Fat
Monterey burger	865	57.0	Chicken Fajita Pita	277	8.0
Large French fries	353	19.0	Side salad	51	3.0
32 oz. carbonated			1 Tbsp. low-cal dressing	15	.1
beverage	384	0	Diet carbonated		
			beverage or	0	0
			Carbonated beverage,		
			20 ounces	2	0
Total Calories	1602	76.0	Total Calories	334	11.1
Approx. % calories			Approx. % calories		
from fat	43%		from fat	30%	

JACK-IN-THE-BOX

Instead of That . . .			Try This!		
	Calories	Fat		Calories	Fat
Chicken Supreme			Club Pita	277	8.0
Sandwich	575	36.0	Hot chocolate	133	4.0
Onion rings	382	23.0			
Iced tea, with sugar	60	59.0			
Total Calories	987	59	Total Calories	410	12.0
Approx. % calories			Approx. % calories		
from fat	54%		from fat	26%	

JACK-IN-THE-BOX BREAKFAST

Instead of That . . .			Try This!		
	Calories	Fat		Calories	Fat
Pancake platter	630	27.0	Breakfast Jack, no egg	227	9.0
Coffee with cream and			Coffee	0	0
sugar	37	1.6			
Total Calories	667	28.6	Total Calories	227	9.0
Approx. % calories			Approx. % calories		
from fat	39%		from fat	28%	

KENTUCKY FRIED CHICKEN

Instead of That . . .	Calories	Fat	Try This!	Calories	Fat
Breast, center, crispy	353	20.9	Breast, center, new lite		
Biscuit	269	13.6	recipe	257	7.0
French fries	268	12.8	Mashed potatoes and		
Corn on the cob	176	3.1	gravy	103	3.0
Total Calories	1066	50.4	Total Calories	360	10.0
Approx. % calories			Approx. % calories		
from fat	43%		from fat	25%	

McDONALD'S BREAKFAST

Instead of That . . .	Calories	Fat	Try This!	Calories	Fat
Biscuit with sausage and			Egg McMuffin, no egg	257	9.4
egg	585	39.9	Coffee	0	0
Hash brown potatoes	125	7.0			
Coffee, cream, and sugar	97	1.6			
Total Calories	807	48.5	Total Calories	257	9.4
Approx. % calories			Approx. % calories		
from fat	54%		from fat	33%	

WENDY'S

Instead of That . . .	Calories	Fat	Try This!	Calories	Fat
Big Classic Double			Chili, reg.	240	8.0
Cheeseburger	780	39.0	6 Saltine crackers	78	1.8
Large French fries	403	19.5	Tea	0	0
Large Frosty dairy					
dessert	680	18.2			
Total Calories	1863	76.7	Total Calories	318	9.8
Approx. % calories			Approx. % calories		
from fat	37%		from fat	28%	

TRY THESE TRIGGER, COMFORT, SNACK, AND JUNK FOODS

Instead of That . . .	Try This!
1 slice regular cheesecake	**1 slice Classic Cheesecake** (see page 221 for recipe)

Instead of That . . .			Try This!		
1 slice regular cheesecake			**1 slice Classic Cheesecake** (see page 221 for recipe)		
Calories	Grams of Fat	% of Fat	Calories	Grams of Fat	% of Fat
309	18	52	103	2	16
			1 slice Pineapple Cheesecake (see page 222 for recipe)		
			Calories	Grams of Fat	% of Fat
			105	1	8
French fries, large			**Skinny French Fries** (see page 225 for recipe)		
Calories	Grams of Fat	% of Fat	Calories	Grams of Fat	% of Fat
357	18	46	120	2	15
Cheese Ball (made with cheddar, 1.5 oz.)			**Party Cheese Ball** (see page 225 for recipe)		
Calories	Grams of Fat	% of Fat	Calories	Grams of Fat	% of Fat
171	14	74	94	8	74
Nabisco Escort crackers (3)			**Nabisco Wheat Thins (8)**		
Calories	Grams of Fat	% of Fat	Calories	Grams of Fat	% of Fat
80	4	45	70	3	34
Ice cream sundae			**Lowfat and low-cal sundae**		
8 oz. Haagen-Daz chocolate chip			4 oz. ice milk chocolate flavor		
Calories	Grams of Fat	% of Fat	Calories	Grams of Fat	% of Fat
620	36	52	110	2.3	19
4 Tbsp. Hershey chocolate fudge topping			1 Tbsp. sugar-free, no-fat chocolate topping		
Calories	Grams of Fat	% of Fat	Calories	Grams of Fat	% of Fat
190	8	36	20	0	0
1 oz. pecans			⅓ cup fresh strawberries, sliced		
Calories	Grams of Fat	% of Fat	Calories	Grams of Fat	% of Fat
195	19	88	15	0	0
2 Tbsp. whipped cream			2 Tbsp. Lite Cool Whip		
Calories	Grams of Fat	% of Fat			
16	2	84			
Candied cherry					
Calories	Grams of Fat	% of Fat	Calories	Grams of Fat	% of Fat
12	0	0	16	trace	trace
Totals 1033	65	56.1	Totals 161	2.3	13

Instead of That . . .	Try This!
Pillsbury Microwave Popcorn (3 cups) Calories — 192 Grams of Fat — 11.5 % of Fat — 54	**Buttery Popcorn, 3 cups** (see page 226 for recipe) Calories — 108 Grams of Fat — 1.5 % of Fat — 12
Wolf Brand Chili with Beans (1 cup) Calories — 345 Grams of Fat — 22 % of Fat — 57	**Easy Texas Chili and Pintos (1 cup)** (see page 226 for recipe) Calories — 198 Grams of Fat — 3 % of Fat — 14
Coke float 8 oz. vanilla ice cream, premium Calories — 349 Grams of Fat — 23.7 % of Fat — 61 8 oz. Coca-Cola Calories — 103 Grams of Fat — 0 % of Fat — 0 Totals — 442 / 23.7 / 48	**Coke float** 8 oz. ice milk Calories — 184 Grams of Fat — 5.6 % of Fat — 27 8 oz. diet Coca-Cola Calories — 1 Grams of Fat — 0 % of Fat — 0 185 / 5.6 / 27
Grilled cheese sandwich 2 slices commercial bread Calories — 160 Grams of Fat — 2 % of Fat — 11 1 slice American cheese Calories — 106 Grams of Fat — 9 % of Fat — 76 2 tsp. regular margarine, Fleischmann's soft Calories — 67 Grams of Fat — 7.4 % of Fat — 99 Totals — 333 / 18.4 / 50	**Low-Cal Grilled Cheese Sandwich** (see page 230 for recipe) Calories — 150 Grams of Fat — 4.7 % of Fat — 28
Sour cream type dips, flavored, Land O' Lakes (3.4 oz.) Calories — 140 Grams of Fat — 10 % of Fat — 64 **Corn chips (2 oz.)** Calories — 306 Grams of Fat — 8.8 % of Fat — 26	**Ricotta Vegetable Dip (3.4 oz.)** (see page 227 for recipe) Calories — 113 Grams of Fat — 4.25 % of Fat — 34 or **Basic Yogurt Cheese (3.4 oz.)** (see page 227 for recipe) Calories — 81 Grams of Fat — 0 % of Fat — 0

Instead of That . . .	Try This!
	*Vegetable dippers are free foods for everyone. You may also use a lower calorie chip, such as Guiltless Gourmet tostado chips, rice cakes, or Skinny Haven chips. These lower fat chips are usually less than 150 calories for a larger portion. Picante salsa is also a free food.
Brownies, Rainbow (1)	No-Cholesterol Brownies (1) (see page 224 for recipe)

Instead of That — Brownies, Rainbow (1):

Calories	Grams of Fat	% of Fat
230	12	47

Try This — No-Cholesterol Brownies (1):

Calories	Grams of Fat	% of Fat
105	4	34

TRY THESE INGREDIENTS

Instead of That . . .	Calories	Grams of Fat	Try This!	Calories	Grams of Fat
1 Tbsp. butter or margarine	100	11.0	1 Tbsp. diet margarine	50	6.0
			Buttery flavored sprinkles	6	0
2 Tbsp. sour cream	60	5.0	2 Tbsp. light sour cream	40	3.5
			2 Tbsp. puréed cottage cheese	25	1.0
			2 Tbsp. plain nonfat yogurt	12.5	0
1 oz. hard cheese	110	9.0	1 oz. part-skim mozzarella	72	4.5
			1 oz. fat-free, Kraft	45	0
			2 Tbsp. grated Parmesan	46	3.0
1 whole egg	80	6.0	¼ cup egg substitute	25	0
			2 egg whites	20	0
1 cup whole milk	160	9.0	1 cup 2% milk	121	4.7
			1 cup 1% milk	104	2.4
			1 cup skim milk	86	.4
2 Tbsp. regular mayonnaise	200	22.4	2 Tbsp. light mayonnaise	80	6.0
			2 Tbsp. Kraft FREE	24	0
			¼ cup Miracle Whip, Kraft	138	10.0
			¼ cup Miracle Whip, light	88	6.0
			¼ cup plain nonfat yogurt	20	0
1 cup whole milk ricotta cheese	432	32.0	1 cup part skim ricotta	342	19.6
			1 cup regular cottage cheese	217	9.5
			1 cup lowfat cottage cheese	164	2.3
			1 cup dry curd cottage cheese	123	.6
1 cup heavy cream, liquid	832	90.0	1 cup light cream	464	46.4
			1 cup half and half	320	27.2
			1 cup evaporated whole milk	338	4.8
			1 cup evaporated skim milk	200	.8

TRY THESE INGREDIENTS (continued)

Instead of That . . .			Try This!		
	Calories	Grams of Fat		Calories	Grams of Fat
1 cup ice cream	349	23.7	1 cup ice milk	184	5.6
			1 cup sherbet	270	3.8
			1 cup frozen yogurt	200	7.0
			1 cup nonfat yogurt	150	0
			1 cup fruit ice, Haagen-Daz	190	0
1 oz. cream cheese	98	10.0	1 oz. reduced-fat cream cheese	62	4.7
			1 oz. puréed lowfat cottage cheese	41	.6
1 cup white sauce	275	20.0	1 cup lowfat white sauce using:		
			2% milk	121	4.7
			1% milk	104	2.4
			Skim milk	86	.4

HOME COOKIN'

Instead of That . . .	Try This!
Hamburger Helper main dishes (1/5 pkg. with 1/5 ground beef)	**Hamburger Hash** (see page 231 for recipe)

Calories	Grams of Fat	% of Fat
335	15	40

Calories	Grams of Fat	% of Fat
270	8	27

Instead of That . . .	Try This!
Swedish Meat Balls, Armor Dinner Classics	**Swedish Meatballs** (about 6–8 meatball serving) (see page 232 for recipe)

Calories	Grams of Fat	% of Fat
450	28.8	58

Calories	Grams of Fat	% of Fat
215	8.1	34

Instead of That . . .	Try This!
Commercial salad dressings (average, 1 Tbsp.)	**Thousand Island Dressing** (1 Tbsp.) (see page 228 for recipe)

Calories	Grams of Fat	% of Fat
85	9	95

Calories	Grams of Fat	% of Fat
17	0.6	31

Blue Cheese Dressing (1 Tbsp.) (see page 228 for recipe)

Calories	Grams of Fat	% of Fat
27	2	67

Instead of That . . .	Try This!
Vegetable Soup, Campbell's (1 cup)	**Vegetarian Vegetable Soup** (1 cup) (see page 230 for recipe)

Calories	Grams of Fat	% of Fat
79	1.5	17

Calories	Grams of Fat	% of Fat
25	0.2	7

Instead of That . . .	Try This!
Chicken Enchiladas, El Charrito (2)	**Chicken Enchiladas Verdes** (2) (see page 233 for recipe)

Calories	Grams of Fat	% of Fat
300	13	40

Calories	Grams of Fat	% of Fat
250	4.4	16

Salsa Verde (1 Tbsp.) (see page 234 for recipe)

Calories	Grams of Fat	% of Fat
6	0.1	2

Instead of That . . .	Try This!
Spinach and Onion Quicke, Pour a Quiche	**Spinach Quiche** (see page 231 for recipe)

Calories	Grams of Fat	% of Fat
220	16	65

Calories	Grams of Fat	% of Fat
192	9.5	45

HOME COOKIN' (continued)

Instead of That . . .	Try This!
Pumpkin Pie, Banquet (1/6 small) *Calories* *Grams of Fat* *% of Fat* 197 8 37	**Thanksgiving Pumpkin Pie (1 serving)** (see page 224 for recipe) *Calories* *Grams of Fat* *% of Fat* 175 4.7 24
Chicken Club Sandwich, Wendy's *Calories* *Grams of Fat* *% of Fat* 479 25 47	**Club Sandwich** (see page 229 for recipe) *Calories* *Grams of Fat* *% of Fat* 290 5.8 18
Typical hamburger *Calories* *Grams of Fat* *% of Fat* 450 19 38	For a lowfat hamburger, look for light buns in your area that contain only 80 calories for the entire bun. Also, see if your grocer can get Healthy Choice ground round beef. It is the lowest in fat on the market, containing only 130 calories for a three-ounce cooked portion. Combining the 80 calorie bun, 130 calorie beef patty, and few extra calories for condiments, you can see how you can make a hamburger for less than 300 calories.

THE LAST WORD

You have had a smattering of the many wonderful ways you can cut fat out of your diet both at home and while eating out. If you stick with your basic premises of knowing which foods inherently contain fat and which do not, easy decision making will become commonplace and routine.

Set Your Mind upon Change

I had not seen Joyce Crane for more than five years. As she walked in, I hoped she didn't notice that I instinctively winced when it became clear how much weight she had regained. When I first met Joyce, she had just turned thirty and was looking introspectively at her life, as most of us do when we pass into a new decade. She had always struggled with her weight, but now she was tipping the scales at 280 pounds—more than twice what her frame should have carried for her height. Her marriage of seven years had ended in divorce. She did not have children, nor did she want them.

She had been a nutrition patient of mine several years ago, before I began working with the *Love Hunger* material. She had actually done quite well. At one time she was down to 170 pounds. She had followed an innovative weight-loss program she thought would remain with her for life. And, now five years later, she was in my office again, looking for new answers to the same old question.

I sent Joyce home with a copy of *Love Hunger* and *The Love Hunger Weight-Loss Workbook*. We were planning for her to join a *Love Hunger* support group as soon as her schedule allowed. In the next few weeks, she devoured the information in the books instead of the comfort foods she had come to depend upon. By the time she came to the first group session, she had already lost fourteen pounds.

We came to find out that Joyce had been adopted, as had her brother. Her parents were older when they began the adoption process and were a little "set in their ways" when they entered into parenthood. Joyce described them as intolerant and somewhat aloof. She always tried to be the "good kid," since her brother was so rebellious. Eventually, being a mascot and "the girl with the funny personality" worked for her, both at home and at school. (To this day, Joyce is a delightful, gregarious woman who is fun to be with.)

When that first layer of laughter was peeled back, though, a much different story began to emerge. Joyce had many deep hurts that had never been addressed. As an adult, she began searching for her biological parents. Joyce found that her birth mother had died several years previously, and there was no record of who her father might have been. That was a bitter pill for her to swallow. I think Joyce was hoping that there could be some sort of bonding with her biological parents, since she didn't feel a love bond with her adoptive parents.

CHOOSE LIFE

Joyce continued to do well, and by the end of only eleven weeks she had lost nearly forty pounds (you can do that at these higher weights). Beyond the physical changes, however, mental changes were also occurring. At one key session Joyce told us, "I always did a good job of covering up what I was really feeling. I even made fat people jokes. Sure, they hurt, but at least I could rest in the fact that people were laughing with me instead of at me. Just like it says in the *Love Hunger Workbook*, compulsive eating is a slow form of suicide. That's just exactly what I was doing! I know it is! Although it's still hard to imagine, I think a few months ago I suddenly woke up, and now I want to live. I am desperate for life, in fact. But I have all these nasty little habits and behaviors from a lifetime of self-abuse with food. Habits like picking up a meal to eat in the car on the way home from work, when I know that I am going out to dinner with friends. Or grabbing up two or three candy bars at a time at the gas station, just as payment to myself for making a long car trip alone.

Or telling myself I won't eat anything the next day, just because I blew it the day before. I want to be nice to myself for the rest of my life. I am entitled to happiness just as much as anyone else."

The rest of the group was dumbfounded at Joyce's clear insight. We went on to assure her—and each other—that after our basic needs are met, we can then attack these habits for what they are, behaviors. Generally, a behavior can be substantially changed in just a few months. I am not going to tell you that certain foods won't taste good anymore. But your food preferences and portion sizes can truly change in a relatively short time, even as little as two months. Once you have found that you desperately want life, as Joyce does, you can find the strength to change those things that are temporal.

Let's quickly review the cycle of food addiction that can result from *love hunger*.

ADDICTION TO FOOD IS A POSSIBILITY

The definition of an addict is someone who is "habitually devoted or surrendered to something." The key element in this definition is not the object of the devotion. Instead, it is the devotion itself, the total surrender to that object at all costs; and the reason for that devotion. What emptiness or void does that devotion fill, which is not being met in other ways in our lives? These important questions must be asked in our world of so many unhappy, addicted people.

One of my patients was a hard-charging businessman who told me he had given up smoking and drinking at the urgent request of his doctor. In fact, he had completed the Alcoholics Anonymous program. One of his revealing statements to me was, "Now I eat like I used to smoke and drink."

You can see from his statement that you can actually be addicted to many things, of which food may be only one. We are all familiar with addictions to substances, such as alcohol and drugs. But we can also be addicted to behaviors, such as compulsive eating, shopping, shoplifting, overachieving, television watching, or using pornography. There is even such a thing as addiction to relationships, which we now call codependency.

Do you think you are addicted to food? Look at the Food Addiction Inventory below, and see how many of the questions you would answer with a yes.

1. Do you eat when you are angry?   Yes _____   No _____
2. Do you eat to comfort yourself in times of crisis or tension?
   Yes _____   No _____
3. Do you eat to stave off boredom?   Yes _____   No _____
4. Do you lie to yourself and others about how much you have eaten or when you ate?   Yes _____   No _____
5. Do you hide food away for yourself?   Yes _____   No _____
6. Are you embarrassed about your physical appearance?
   Yes _____   No _____
7. Are you 20 percent or more over your medically recommended weight?   Yes _____   No _____
8. Have significant people in your life expressed concern about your eating pattern?   Yes _____   No _____
9. Has your weight fluctuated by more than ten pounds in the past six months?   Yes _____   No _____
10. Do you fear that your eating is out of control?   Yes _____   No _____

If you answer positively to even a few of these questions, you probably have some emotional ties with food that could be considered a food addiction.

The bottom line is this: What are your motivations? Are your daily actions based on legitimate human needs? Or are you trying to cover up pain from your past or present situations? Are you numbing the hurt instead of dealing with it? What are you a slave to? Is food an answer on the list of possibilities?

SIX STEPS TO ADDICTION

I realize that many of you have read the other *Love Hunger* books previously to this third in the series. For those who haven't read the first two books; I feel compelled to spend a few pages on the basic concepts that were the hallmarks of those books. (Those who are familiar with this material may want to skim the next few pages or skip them entirely.)

Below is shown the six-step downward spiral developed by the Love Hunger program. See how you might fit into this cycle.

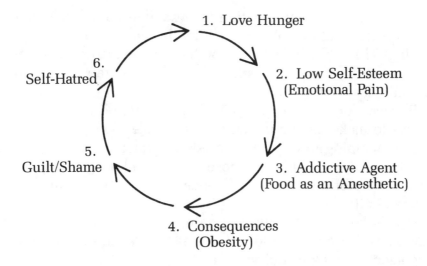

1. Love Hunger

2. Low Self-Esteem
(Emotional Pain)

3. Addictive Agent
(Food as an Anesthetic)

4. Consequences
(Obesity)

5. Guilt/Shame

6. Self-Hatred

Step One: Love Hunger

Many people go through life with a love deficit, what we call love hunger. Sometimes this can simply translate into unmet needs, perhaps as a result of coming from a dysfunctional family—such as a family where one or both parents had addiction problems. Or it may stem from problems arising in adulthood, such as a difficult marriage, divorce, death of a loved one, several job-related problems, or a debilitating illness.

Step Two: Low Self-Esteem

One of the results of love hunger is a loss of self-esteem. Having been given the message that we are unworthy, we believe it (especially if we are told this as a child). Now we live under an ominous cloud, waiting for it to burst at any second.

Nothing we do seems right. If everyone else thinks we're worthless, well, maybe we are. If our spouse or parents have told us how terrible we are, shouldn't we believe them? Sometimes we seem to experience precious little evidence or reassurance to the contrary.

Step Three: Addictive Agent

As the pain associated with this low self-esteem develops, most people are tempted to look for anything that can cover up its venomous sting. Think of the last time you had a serious toothache or nausea. You knew you needed help and wanted to grab the first thing that could ease the pain.

Believe it or not, we willingly choose addictive agents. We look for ways to make the emotional pain bearable. Some choose work, food, or shopping to take their minds off those things that are too painful to deal with. Others choose alcohol and drugs, perhaps due to easy accessibility and the influence of others, including the immediate family.

Is this how you handle the pain in your life? Wouldn't you rather be healed once and for all, instead of depending on anesthetizing agents for the rest of your life?

Step Four: Consequences

The consequences of unwise actions invariably surface. These repercussions can range anywhere from increasing your clothing size to losing your home, your family, or your life. Often, it is only at this stage that we begin to take action. When the doctor finally says, "Lose weight or die," it's time to take that diet seriously.

I know you have heard this lecture too many times, but obesity can increase your chances of heart disease, cancer, and diabetes—the major killers of Americans. Are you prepared to accept these consequences?

Step Five: Guilt and Shame

Most addiction is initially driven by shame. And now, with the food addiction firmly in place, the shame is confirmed and even re-affirmed in your own mind. Now the old shame that stemmed from our low self-esteem and the new shame from being an addict work together to compound our addiction.

If this is the point you are at right now, keep these important truths in mind. The past is the past. The future is still beyond our reach. We can only control what happens today. We can always make a fresh start.

Step Six: Self-Hatred

It is easy to see how self-hatred and even self-destruction are often the last step in this cycle. This self-hatred can add even more fuel to the fire. Now we have to deal with self-scorn as well as scorn from others.

THE FIVE GREATEST EMOTIONAL PITFALLS FOR DIETERS

Emotional recovery is not as simple as an overstretched rubber band popping back into place. It takes time, effort, and work to shed that extra emotional baggage we've been lugging around. In fact, learning who we are and why we are as we are may be one of the single greatest challenges in life. Contentment with self and how you fit into the world around you stills the mind, nurtures the soul, and usually aids in dieting success.

My clinical work with individual patients has allowed me to view human motivation and contentment at a very intimate level. For example, perhaps someone comes to my office because they have elevated serum lipid levels (cholesterol and triglycerides) and were sent by their physician. Within thirty minutes, we have discussed a lowfat and low-cholesterol diet. Then we move into the area of weight loss. On their next visit, we talk about why they did or did not stick with their prescribed diet for the week. For some, who are unencumbered with all the extra emotional baggage, things go well; they lose weight, and their blood levels usually normalize.

But others just never seem to get started. As the weeks progress, several recurrent themes seem to emerge that act as negatives and keep these people imprisoned within bad eating habits. The five greatest pitfalls for dieters are blaming offenders, making excuses, not tapping into a higher power, not recognizing the complex nature of weight loss, and not seeking satisfaction in life. As we review these five pitfalls, try to determine if any of these negative issues might be playing out in your own life.

1. *Blaming Offenders*

Internalizing true forgiveness is one of the most difficult things you will ever do. Many of my patients have done well on a diet until ugly issues from the past resurface and bring with them old, formerly suppressed feelings. I have heard about child abuse, sexual molestation, murder, rape, emotional abuse, infidelity, and betrayal from my patients. The real question remains: After these things happen in your life, will you let go of them or will they cause you crippling pain for the rest of your life?

To let go of the pain, we must first learn to successfully and completely grieve. The five stages of successful grieving (talked about in detail in the last two *Love Hunger* books) include (1) shock and denial, (2) anger, (3) bargaining, (4) sadness, and finally (5) acceptance, forgiveness, and resolution. I have had many patients who have book-learned these five steps only to find that they are not yet prepared to make that jump to total forgiveness. Let me tell you about one of them.

Sandra was a single college student who had moved to my city from South Carolina to get away from a past of sexual abuse. She had been sexually abused by an older cousin from the age of seven through high school. When she started realizing that this was not the way everyone lived, she found that other female members of her family had also been abused.

Sandra had been in my weight-loss program for about three months while under pastoral counseling care at the church she attended. When she decided to return to her home for a weeklong winter vacation, I sensed that she was doing so to test herself in some way. You see, when Sandra had told her parents that the sexual abuse had been going on for years, they accused her of making up the whole story. It was perhaps this part of the tragedy that hurt her the most. Now she was not only the victim, but the black sheep of the family.

Sandra had lost nearly twenty pounds before going on her trip. But when she returned, I sensed a change in her demeanor. The anger and resentment had resurfaced because she had never really forgiven her family. The old feelings of shame were resurfacing, and self-doubt was setting in. These insecurities caused her to gain five pounds in the next month.

One day I suggested to Sandra, "I want to draw you a picture of what you are doing to yourself. Imagine that you are on a large lake, fishing in a small boat. You have several fishing lines overboard, and they all have big fish on the hooks. The waves in the lake make things exciting. Some are a little bigger than you anticipated, but things are in control. You have good balance, yet you are becoming weary holding all the fishing lines with large fish on the hooks. You realize that if you could just let go of the strings and let the fish swim away, then you could relax and feel the breeze on your face. The day is beautiful and is meant to be enjoyed. But somehow you just can't because you are burdened with these heavy fishing hooks."

I went on to say, "Sandra, can you see how our lives can be like this? We hold onto those hurts just like we hold onto the fishing lines. It makes staying afloat difficult at best and deadly at worst. It can literally drag us to the bottom. And yet we do it anyway. Life is fun, and you're missing it! What did Rosalind Russell say in Auntie Mame? 'Life is a banquet and most poor suckers are starving to death'? Maybe that's what we are doing when we hang onto those hurts."

The picture below is like the one I drew for Sandra. Can you see yourself in any of this? Do you have hurts in your life that are trying to pull you under? If so, attach names to the fish on the hooks and prepare to let them swim away.

Sandra questioned me at this point, "How can I simply forget that these people have just about ruined my life? Where's the justice in all this?"

At this point I passed her the tissue box and said, "Sandra, the only person who is continuing to suffer from all this is you. And every time you wince from the pain of it all, you are the victim once again.

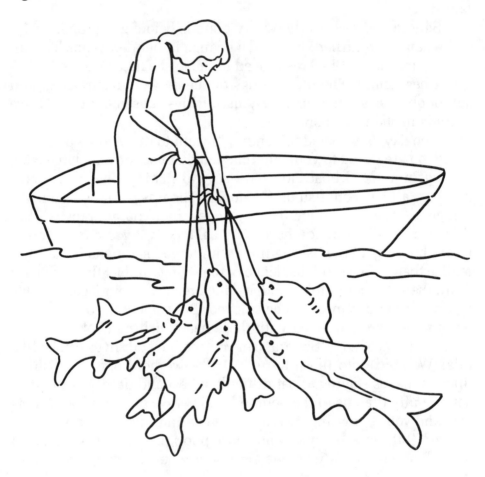

"Are you still under the delusion that this world is fair? Nothing could be further from the truth. All you have to do to prove inequities and unfairness is to pick up any newspaper."

I continued, "But I've got to say this too. Just because victims let the bad guys off the hook doesn't mean that they are off of God's hook. The hook is still in their mouths; you're just not holding onto them anymore." Since Sandra was a Christian, I suggested that we think about forgiveness in light of her beliefs. "Look at the wisdom in this verse from the Bible," I said.

If someone wrongs you, do not pay him back by doing wrong to him. Try to do what everyone thinks is right. Do your best to live in peace with everyone. My friends, do not try to punish others when they wrong you. Wait for God to punish them with his anger. It is written: "I am the One who punishes; I will pay people back," says the Lord. (Romans 12:17–19, International Children's Version Bible)

"Okay," said Sandra, "That makes sense to me. I think I really can forgive, but how do I forget?" I then told her, "Believe it or not, I don't want you to forget. Leave it on the back burner? Sure. But while the memories are becoming dim, perhaps you can take solace in a quote from Dr. Paul Meier, 'Forgiveness is not excusing, or tolerating, or justifying, which are ways that we frequently try to cope with having been wronged. Nor is it minimizing the pain. Forgiveness is an act of the will, just like happiness is a choice. We choose to forgive others because God forgives our sins.'"[5]

Are there fishing lines in your own life? Do they need to be dropped so you can get on with things? If so, make a list of whom you need to forgive for hurting you, what you need to forgive yourself for, and whose forgiveness you need to seek. Remember, this is not an emotional exercise, but an act of the will. Tear up that list, drop the fishing hooks and lines, and start your diet (and perhaps your life) again. Look for smooth sailing.

2. *Making Excuses*

Excuse making, rationalizing, defending, justifying, and explaining away poor health habits and dietary indiscretions has to go. There is no way around this monster but to serve it a deathblow.

Now don't get me wrong about this. Perfection is still not required. But honesty is. Dietary honesty means that when you make less than optimal choices, you clearly identify the problem and begin taking corrective measures so this will happen less frequently. It also means that you are taking full responsibility for your actions instead of blaming poor choices you have made on someone else or difficult circumstances around or about you.

Let's get specific and look at some actual excuses that might keep us from doing our best in revitalizing our health.

It's hard for me to lose weight. Everyone in my family is obese. Why should I expect myself to be any different? Maybe I should just be fat and happy!

This is a toughy, and one that I have struggled with myself. Obesity does seem to be genetic. But so do big brown eyes, athletic ability, musical talent, high blood pressure, diabetes, some cancers, and even personality. All of us are a composite of desirable, and perhaps less than desirable, traits by today's value system. Our mission in life is not to lament what we do not have, though, but to optimize what we do have. Remember this, there hasn't been a perfect human being since Adam and Eve, and even they managed to blow it.

I have heard many a frustrated dieter proclaim that diets just don't work for them. And that they have, therefore, decided to give up trying. They also say that the real worth of the person is on the inside and has nothing to do with the outside appearance and that they feel totally justified in status quo obesity.

I've just got to throw the flag on that one, friends. I know that it is your character and soul that make you who you are. But if you are more than forty pounds overweight (or greater than 30 percent of your ideal weight), can you honestly tell me that it doesn't make you less effective in your daily life?

We're talking honesty here. Does it not affect your relationship with your spouse in some way? Does it not affect your own feelings of sexuality? Does it not affect your level of patience with children or others who require your attention? When was the last time you were overly harsh and critical of your kids because you had a lousy dieting day? Does it keep you from going to social gatherings where you feel uncomfortable about your appearance? Does it keep you from being assertive about your true feelings for fear of being ridiculed?

Please don't get mad and slam this book closed. I have had enough experience with my own weight concerns and that of hundreds of other patients to know that these are genuine and often unspoken hurts. They are usually the type of hurts you feel you can't tell anyone. Things you go in the shower to cry about where no one else can know the depth of your despair. Starting today, don't gloss over these things and say that everything is okay. Likewise, don't hide behind a shield that says "I can't." The fact is, you *can* lose that weight and change your health status for the rest of your life, regardless of your genetic makeup.

"I have too much hurt in my life to be successful in dieting right now. Maybe I can work on this later."

At a seminar I once gave in Utah, a woman was concerned about the special consideration that the *Love Hunger* programs give to those who have been emotionally hurt. She was specifically worried that would-be dieters and seminar participants might use these former abuses as excuses for not dieting. She put it this way, "I don't want anything else in my life that could be a crutch or a way for me to evade healthy habits. I have plenty of those already. You're telling us, Dr. Sneed, that we need to first understand our past and present relationships and accept who we are. Well, I've already done that, but I still need to lose weight." I really had to concede that she had made a good point.

In fact, I can even think of a few patients who might fit into this particular category of denial. One forty-year-old former patient began her diet program full of exciting expectations, but also with a sense of uneasiness since it had been quite some time since she had lost weight. After all of the issues of her childhood sexual abuse had been discussed in detail with both me and the patient's other counselor, we all thought that her dietary efforts would flourish. But they did not.

It became my personal opinion that this woman was hiding behind the former abuses to cover up bad habits, which she just simply did not want to change. Any successful dieter must learn a certain amount of delayed gratification. For example, giving up five hundred calories worth of your normal daily food allotment over a six-week period of time to achieve a smaller dress size. You put off a few of the taste sensations and pleasures right now to enjoy a smaller size later on.

I want to stay just short of suggesting that some formerly abused people may be emotionally coddled by their family and even therapists in some compensatory fashion. But are you hiding behind memories from the past so that you can satisfy your behavioral desires for food? Are you avoiding what you should do because you are trying to make up for something that was done to you or is part of your present life? Choose reality. Choose delayed gratification. Choose to be a size smaller next month.

> *I could do better on a diet if only I had more time and less responsibilities.*

There's no mistaking the truth in this common statement. For persons who are genetically more resistant to weight loss than others or those who have a lot of changes to make, your new healthy lifestyle program has to take close to top priority. There must be adequate time for food planning, exercise, and good mental health (a little down time, relaxation).

When you are an overly busy person, it is easy to justify skipping that one-hour workout or grabbing the first edible thing you see for your five-minute lunch. Choices must be made. And sometimes they are very tough ones. Ask yourself if you really have time for everything in your life right now, plus a minimum of an hour per day for your own needs. If this time is not there, are you prepared to give up something?

Some dieters can feel totally justified in their overcommitment if it revolves around one of two things: family or livelihood. Mothers who devote every waking moment to their families are noble indeed. But how long can you keep up this pace? Others, who ask themselves to spend over fifty hours per week working to make a living for their family, also may have good intentions. But is it not better to live more closely within one's means rather than become unhealthy and perhaps cut years off your life?

In a seminar Dr. Robert Hemfelt and I conducted in Austin, Texas, Dr. Hemfelt eloquently addressed this very issue when he said, "Consider the last time you were on an airplane. The stewardess starts giving emergency information as the plane taxis down the runway. You have heard the same little speech many times and tune it out. This trip is different, though. You have your small child beside you in the next seat. Then you wonder, if the cabin really lost pressure and the masks really drop from the ceiling of the plane, would I really put mine on first—before my own child? I would submit to you that if you do not take care of your own safety first, you might black out before the oxygen mask is securely fitted over your child, in which case you both might perish."[6]

We must be well ourselves before we can help anyone else. Take care of yourself, take time for yourself, put fitness near the top of your daily agenda, and you will be amazed how everything else falls into place.

3. Not Tapping into a Higher Power

A good friend and former patient (who has lost thirty pounds and reached her goal weight) once sent me a humorous Valentine's card that completely describes the perpetual dieter who has never found the will to diet. The card shows the cartoon version of a portly woman framed inside a pink heart. She has a rather smug and resolute look on her face. The caption reads, "For years, I've tried to figure out why I sit around on Valentine's Day wolfing chocolate by the pound. I finally got to the root of the problem." And, on the inside of the card, it simply says, "I like wolfing chocolate by the pound."

After you have cut the extra emotional baggage loose, after you have let everyone and everything off your hook, the bad eating habits established by love hunger may still remain. Now is a time when many dieters continue to eat because it is a learned and enjoyable habit. Who will deny that a certain amount of food indulgence doesn't taste good from time to time? Food is intended to be pleasurable to humans. Why else would we have taste buds and experience an endorphin surge after a meal? The key seems to be our willingness to change long-standing habits and develop a new lifestyle.

Any skilled therapist will tell you that until you decide to do something for yourself, no one can talk you into it. Sure, you could be locked away and forced to quit smoking, spending, or binge eating. But what good would that do? As soon as you were released you would resume former behaviors unless you had changed your mind. Until you have firmly established your priorities, permanent change of anything just will not become reality.

I've had dozens of patients just like our obese friend in the Valentine's card—people who think the act of purchasing a book, joining a group, or seeing a nutritionist will provide all the will they need for dieting success. They don't want to change their diet, lifestyle, or anything else; and yet they expect to enjoy weight loss and improved health.

I remember one patient who sat across from my desk and told me in defiance, "But I don't like lowfat milk," when I suggested that whole milk was out of the question for her particular health profile. Even after I assured her that this was something she would get used to, she resisted this and other lifestyle changes. I really wanted to ask her why she was wasting my time and hers.

Folks, there's no getting around the fact that whatever you have been doing in the past is not working: You are going to have to give up a few things, make a few changes, and develop new behaviors.

What if our chocolate eater in the Valentine's card had said, "For years, I've tried to figure out why I sit around wolfing beer and wine. I finally got to the root of the problem. I like wolfing beer and wine." How would we feel if our chocolate compadre were an alcoholic? Is it any less painful if our addiction is overeating, a more socially acceptable addiction? I don't think so.

Changing your lifestyle is a conscious decision you must make. Sure, I can tell you all day long that within six weeks you'll like lowfat milk and enjoy light versions of pizza and meatloaf more than their higher fat alternatives. I can even tell you that your appetite will change and that you will be happy with much smaller amounts of food within four weeks. I can emphasize the absolute joy that comes with seeing your own body at its best. But until you internalize the information and believe that you want this more than the "old ways," no one can help you. You call the shots.

In the previous two *Love Hunger* books, we used the Twelve-Step program of Overeater's Anonymous. The steps are listed again below. Keep in mind that our other books have given extensive discussion of these Steps and you may refer to them for more depth.

The thing to keep in mind is that willpower requires effort on your part as well as empowerment by God. You must decide you will do this—nothing can substitute for that determination. After you have made that choice, you may then ask God to help you stay with the program and give you strength to carry on. Read on in the next section for more information on tapping into God's higher power.

1. We admitted we were powerless over our dependencies—that our lives had become unmanageable. 2. Came to believe that a Power greater than ourselves could restore us to sanity. 3. Made a decision to turn our will and our lives over to the care of God, as we understood Him. 4. Made a searching and fearless moral inventory of ourselves. 5. Admitted to God, to ourselves, and to another human being the exact nature of our wrongs. 6. Were entirely ready to have God remove all these defects of character. 7. Humbly asked Him to remove our shortcomings. 8. Made a list of all persons we had harmed and became willing to make amends to them all. 9. Made direct amends to such people wherever possible, except when to do so would injure them or others. 10. Continued to take personal inventory and when we were wrong, promptly admitted it. 11. Sought through prayer and meditation to improve our conscious contact with God, praying only for knowledge of His will for us and the power to carry that out. 12. Having had a spiritual awakening as the result of these steps, we tried to carry this message to others, and to practice these principles in all our affairs.

THE TWELVE STEPS OF ALCOHOLICS ANONYMOUS

1. We admitted we were powerless over alcohol—that our lives had become unmanageable. 2. Came to believe that a Power greater than ourselves could restore us to sanity. 3. Made a decision to turn our will and our lives over to the care of God as we understood Him. 4. Made a searching and fearless moral inventory of ourselves. 5. Admitted to God, to ourselves and to another human being the exact nature of our wrongs. 6. Were entirely ready to have God remove all these defects of character. 7. Humbly asked Him to remove our shortcomings. 8. Made a list of all persons we had harmed, and became willing to make amends to them all. 9. Made direct amends to such people

wherever possible, except when to do so would injure them or others. 10. Continued to take personal inventory and when we were wrong promptly admitted it. 11. Sought through prayer and meditation to improve our conscious contact with God, as we understood Him, praying only for knowledge of His will for us and the power to carry that out. 12. Having had a spiritual awakening as the result of these steps, we tried to carry this message to alcoholics, and to practice these principles in all our affairs.

4. Not Recognizing the Complex Nature of Weight Loss

I would like you to look at the drawing on the next page. Can you see how many factors are involved in the careful scheme of weight loss? I envision it like this. The circle on page 115 represents our whole being as it relates to weight loss. Armor surrounds, adjoins, unites, and even protects all the various subareas. When you are fulfilling the requirements (or most of them) within each subarea, weight-loss and weight-maintenance success follow. At this point you are usually balanced and generally happy. When there is a breakdown in one area, though, it is more difficult to maintain and protect your perimeters. And just like a piece of fruit, when decay begins in one small area, the whole piece can literally rot from the inside out. (Luckily, we can always start afresh with a new piece of fruit.)

Physical

Eating behaviors. Developing good eating habits about where, when, and how much you eat is an essential. Proper plate size, rate of eating, style of eating, and your eating place can save hundreds of indiscriminately eaten calories per day.

Activity levels. Most authorities agree that you must be willing to change exercise/fitness/activity levels, or no diet will ever be successful. During maintenance, walking three miles per day can allow you to eat three hundred more calories per day without gaining weight (see chapter 7).

Heredity. Up to 65 percent of obesity is an inherited trait. But everyone inherits both positive and negative characteristics. Focus on those things that are indeed gifts within your own self, and know that anyone can be at their ideal weight with patience and effort.

Cooking habits. Changing your methods and style of cooking can save you hundreds of unneeded calories per day without sacrificing anything to taste (see previous *Love Hunger* books and chapter 4).

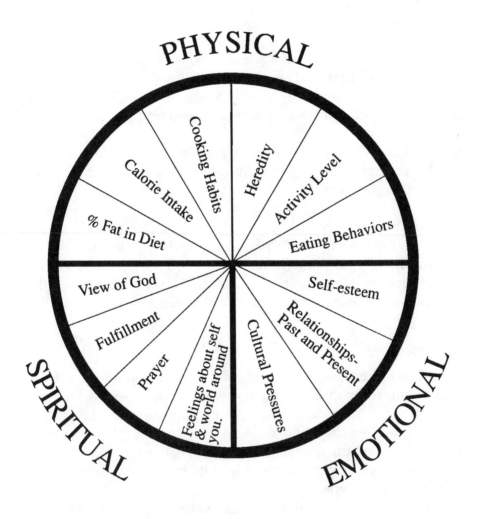

The Whole You and Obesity

Calorie intake. Calorie intake must come down in a weight-loss program. But most people feel that a well-balanced, twelve-hundred calorie diet is more food than they were eating in the first place.

Percent of calories as fat in daily diet. We should aim at lowering our overall dietary fat intake to 25 percent or less of the caloric intake as fat. This by itself is a huge step toward dietary success.

Emotional

Self-esteem. Though not a major focus of this book, this is discussed in detail in the other *Love Hunger* books. People who do not feel good about themselves usually are not successful in dieting. If this applies, find out what is bothering you and put it to rest.

Relationships—past and present. Care must be taken to be honest with yourself and to discover if there is love hunger in your own life. (See page 120.)

Cultural pressures. Don't let anyone in your life talk you into eating food you really don't like. Nor should you let them tell you that you must find contentment in remaining fifty pounds overweight because others around you are in the same situation. Misery loves company, and they will feel challenged if you go on a diet.

Spiritual

Some of you may be surprised to find a traditionally trained doctor of nutrition and registered dietitian like myself talking about the connection between your spiritual nature and weight loss. In fact it should not be surprising at all considering that the most widely accepted addiction recovery program in the world, Alcoholics Anonymous, also defers to and bases its entire program on getting help from "the Higher Power."

Who would deny that inappropriate eating is also an addiction? Think of the last time you tried to keep yourself from eating something you really wanted. Were you successful in stopping the destructive behavior? Or did you feel powerless to overcome the temptation?

Some will say that all you need is more willpower. Well, what exactly is that and how do you get it? My definition of willpower is this, you supply the will and let God supply the power. If you could summarize the essence of any Twelve-Step program, it might be just that. In the course of changing and maintaining this new lifestyle, use prayer and communion with God as your strength—especially when you have none left to give.

My own Higher Power is the God of the Bible and His Son Jesus Christ. He is forgiving, loving, and knows every detail of my life and yours. He is patient, knows my cares and worries, and, believe it or not, has everything under control in an eternal perspective.

Some of you are undoubtedly thinking at this point, "Can I use this book if I am an atheist, agnostic, member of another faith, or just never thought about it?" Absolutely is my answer to you. Beyond a listing of the twelve steps of Overeater's Anonymous, the rest of the book deals with more physical issues and tangible subjects like what kind of frozen desserts to buy at the supermarket and how to make a 150-calorie grilled cheese sandwich. But if you have never thought about God or have closed Him out of your life for a long time, I offer you this verse from the Old Testament: "But from there you will seek the LORD your God, and you will find Him if you seek Him with all your heart and with all your soul" (Deut. 4:29 NKJV).

5. *Not Seeking Satisfaction in Life*

All of us have known someone who has every reason on earth to be happy about life—and, sadly, is not. Maybe you are one of these. Perhaps someone close to you is discontented. Beyond the major life issues that have been discussed above there are a few other issues we must address.

If you have been sad and depressed, losing sleep, and suffering with what seems to be an inordinate amount of anxiety for an extended period of time, see a medical doctor to determine if there are any underlying medical conditions that are at present being ignored in stiff-upper-lip fashion.

Clinical depression is a distinct possibility if you fit this description. But it must be determined if this is a temporary thing that has been triggered by a major life event (death of spouse, divorce, bankruptcy) or if this is something that is inherent to your makeup or runs in your family. In either case, help is available.

I have yet to see an untreated depressed person who is able to successfully stay on a weight-loss diet. Depression is not to be considered a moral weakness—or an excuse. You must seek medical help for depression and then look for dietary success as a follow-up. More than clinical depression can cause us to lose satisfaction, however. Let's look at what's required for happy adults.

WHAT ADULTS NEED OUT OF LIFE

In 1963 Eric Erickson was the first to systematically examine the psychological development of individuals over their entire life span. In Erickson's model, each stage of development is distinguished by a specific issue that seems universally important for that stage of life. This information has been corroborated in review material from the American Academy of Family Practice as well. Interestingly, much of this information follows along with the Love Hunger concept, and not completing any of these steps can decrease our satisfaction with ourselves and the world around us.

In the first eighteen months of life, infants learn basic trust or mistrust of themselves and others. If an infant feels love and comfort, this will usually develop into a feeling of trust. Through three years of age toddlers will either learn autonomy or shame and doubt. This usually depends on how parents handle failure experiences. From age three to six, young children are beginning to take their parents' ways and rules to heart. Initiative is developing, but children can be made to feel guilty during this phase as well. From ages six to twelve and as the child enters school, everyone's focus turns toward productivity and development of social skills. During this stage a sense of industry (instead of inadequacy) develops in children who are doing well in school and getting along with their peers. During the puberty and adolescence years, self-identity begins to take shape. A consistent, continuous personality and self-concept is something the adolescent must actively pursue.

At this point we have finally reached young adulthood. The unfortunate thing is that if any of these stages were inadequately passed, without meeting all needs, the hesitations, guilt, and self-doubt can carry with you until you, as a willing adult, admit that they are false.

During the young adulthood years, either intimacy or isolation is chosen as a way of life. Intimacy in relationships will bring real happiness. Intimacy is defined as the ability to develop and maintain close, enduring relationships. In most cases, these relationships require compromise and self-sacrifice. The old adolescent peer group begins to lose some of its glamour during this stage of intimacy as courtship, marriage, and lifelong friendships emerge.

I have had numerous obese men and women in my practice who are of the most loving and generous sort, and yet they have no friends. Many overweight persons feel so bad about their body image that they avoid all contact except family. If you find yourself in this category of isolation, break out! You are lovable. Other lonely people who need you are out there right now. Losing the weight has nothing to do with these friendships.

By the time we reach middle adulthood, we all hope to "have our act together." The key seems to be: Are we creating or are we stagnating? Believe it or not, paying the bills and putting food on the table is not good enough. It really is necessary that we enjoy our work and that we have some sort of creative outlet in order to be happy. Erickson also claimed that our work and creativity should take the form of helping others besides ourself. Healthy individuals in this stage nurture others and become invested in their growth rather than only looking after themselves. Those who do not reach this stage of generativity face stagnation or the termination of further psychological development.

It is interesting to observe this particular stage among my weight-loss patients. Once considered something akin to folk medicine, it seems that including acts of generosity and kindness in our daily lives rather than living just for self is truly "just what the doctor ordered." When we focus only on self, nothing is ever good enough and life always falls short of our expectations.

If your life-satisfaction levels are low, ask yourself these questions:

- Do I enjoy my work? Yes _____ No _____
- Am I allowed creativity in my work? Yes _____ No _____
- Do I make time to give part of myself back to others in need? Yes _____ No _____

Can you see how including these major factors in your life could solve some mental problems that may be driving you to eat inappropriately? Keep in mind that weight control can depend on many factors. Find the ones that apply to you, and focus on these issues until they are solved. Shore up that armor and be prepared to approach weight loss as a whole person.

Now let's move on into the realm of behaviors. Did you know that it only takes about six weeks for many of us to change major, lifelong habits? Turn to the next action step to see how your behaviors can be modified.

Adopt Winning Behaviors and Guidelines for Permanent Weight Loss

Weight management is a lifestyle. In order to really make it work, there should be very little "I'm on the diet" or "I'm off the diet" notions. This chapter will help you develop habits that can aid you in your daily decision making. We will talk about behaviors both at home and while eating out. Travel tips and airline meals will also be discussed. Some specific meal choices were given in Action Step 4. Ultimately, I truly believe this: *In every situation, a good nutritional choice can be made.* Keep this axiom in mind, and follow the guidelines below to help you see where problems can be avoided before they ever start.

THE GROUND RULES FOR EATING OUT

1. *Don't approach it haphazardly.* Most people know beforehand when they will be eating out. Plan ahead. Eating out will consistently be the area that will tempt you to eat too many calories. Know which restaurants have good, lowfat choices and which don't. When possible, steer your group away from places where you just can't resist eating too much or where there are no healthy choices to be made.

2. *Plan what types of food you will eat.* Before you look at the menu, decide about how many calories you will eat and what types of foods will complete your day's worth of nutrition. Don't be swayed by an enticing menu; there are usually great-tasting choices to be made in all areas.

3. *Know what you are getting.* Sometimes it is difficult to determine what foods contain. If you are choosing anything that is fried or breaded or has a lot of cheese or heavy sauce or gravy, it is probably not the right choice.

4. *Don't get tricked by large, high-fat salads and soups.* I have observed many restaurant-goers choose a salad (usually with cheese and lots of high-fat dressing) and cheese soup, thinking that they were being prudent. By the time you eat that cheese-laden salad, loaded with oil and vinegar, ranch, blue cheese, or another regular salad dressing, you have probably downed six hundred calories, and that doesn't include the bread, butter, and crackers. Canadian cheese and broccoli soup is another three hundred calories minimum. If you had selected a light dressing or eliminated cheese from the salad and replaced it with cottage cheese or turkey strips, or chosen a clear beef-vegetable soup, the calorie content of the lunch would have been cut in half or even more.

5. *Don't be swayed by friends.* Be the first to order when you are out with a large group of friends. If they make poor and unhealthy choices, you may be tempted to do the same.

6. *Resist partners in crime.* Do you have special friends who have been consistent eating buddies in the past? Do you have a common bond of trying new restaurants and breaking all the rules for that evening? If you had a problem with alcohol, your counselor would tell you that you should not revisit the same old bars, especially with the same old friends. This advice holds true with dieting: just substitute the word *restaurant* for the word *bar*. Don't put yourself into old and uncomfortable situations. Tell your old eating buddies that you still value their friendship but you will have to find a new source of entertainment.

7. *Remember, you're the boss.* Let the restaurant serve you exactly what you want. No skin on chicken? No problem. Dressing on the side? No problem. Salad instead of fries? No problem. Need a take-home carton? No problem.

8. *Say no to extras.* To stay within a calorie intake that will allow you to maintain your weight, eliminate all the restaurant extras— such as special breads, chips, appetizers, desserts, and drinks. Also forgo that large roll with butter, glass of wine, and half serving of dessert, and you will have saved yourself five hundred or more calories added to the total amount of the meal.

9. *Avoid buffets.* I do not recommend that you go to the "all-you-can-eat" restaurants. The temptation to overstuff is too great in an attempt to get your money's worth.

10. *Order à la carte or lowfat appetizers for your main dish.* It is unnecessary to feel forced into ordering a large dinner you really don't want. If you have been dieting, you will usually feel full after a piece of bread and dinner salad. Eight-course dinners have no place in good health maintenance, unless the cuisine is thoughtfully prepared with portion and fat content in mind.

What Foods to Choose in a Restaurant

The guidelines you have established for grocery shopping and choosing foods for yourself should be the same rules you use when eating out. Americans eat out so often that you cannot make reckless decisions simply because you are not in your own kitchen. Getting a "good deal" is not necessarily defined as "getting the most food for your money." Keep your thoughts on long-term goals.

For specific menu recommendations, check the meal comparisons made in Action Step 4.

TRAVEL, BUSINESS, AND AIRPLANE FOOD

I was in the Atlanta airport coming home from a *Love Hunger* book tour when my plane was delayed and I found myself with a few hours to people watch and snoop around the concourse. Having decided that some hot tea and a newspaper would be a nice way to begin my wait, I walked down the crowded aisles to the nearest coffee shop. Several planes had been delayed or canceled that day. Perhaps there was foul weather, I really can't remember.

When I arrived at the smoke-ridden, buffeteria-style coffee shop, it became obvious that I would wait in line a minimum of ten minutes. People were in the aisles, and there was standing room only. Having nothing better to do, I decided to wait my turn.

I noticed a woman who was only two people ahead of me in line. She was about forty-five years old, carried an executive-style briefcase, and had on her business suit with the mandatory one-inch matching pumps and sensible handbag. I could tell that her feet hurt. She looked to be about fifty pounds overweight. This nice-looking, dark-haired woman was obviously on a business trip of some sort and seemed a little tired and frazzled, like she was ready to be home and was dismayed that her plane would be delayed.

Now at this point, you must understand that after having been in the "diet business" for nearly fifteen years I can't help but notice the food choices people make. Whether they are in the grocery store, the table next to me at a restaurant, McDonald's, or the Atlanta airport, I notice who they are, what they choose, and imagine what they are thinking to themselves. Yet I would never make unsolicited advice.

I could sense that this woman was nervous about the food line. She was eyeing several things quickly, her head darting from side to side. She seemed anxious, as if someone would catch her, or perhaps she was subconsciously fearful that the food might run out. Had the line been moving at a quicker pace, I think she could have mustered the courage to get completely through with what she had originally intended to choose. She first chose the chef salad and actually placed it on her tray; but she was looking nervously at the very large brownies (about four inches square), which were on the top shelf of the serving line tray. In a moment, she would have to pass them. They would be within eighteen inches of her nose. Actually, these enormous brownies were only a dollar, a phenomenally cheap price for a traditionally overpriced airport restaurant.

The line inched along as others in front of us purchased their provisions. She was now within arm's reach of the brownies. I noticed her looking around tentatively at other people, other food selections, her watch, her own self. Within the next few seconds the prepackaged salad went back to the serving shelf and the mammoth brownie was placed squarely on her tray. Now she was really struggling, choices had to be made, and there was no turning back. The rest of the world was oblivious to the battle going on inside her head, but I knew what she was struggling against—I had fought this enemy many times myself. Perhaps if I had been standing directly next to her, I might have made a joke about the size of the brownie or tried to help her in some other way. It just wasn't possible though.

The line had been crossed now, so what the heck? She now began to focus on what else she might choose to go with the brownie. She continued putting things on her tray until she had a hamburger (with mayo), a large bag of potato chips (250 calories per bag), a non-dietetic soda, and, of course, the brownie. All in all, I tallied up about 1400 calories on her tray.

As she stepped up to the cashier, she looked surprisingly unhappy for a person who had just indulged every whimsical appetite. Is that how you feel when things like this happen? Perhaps you have gone to a business or social luncheon with good intentions that never materialized. Maybe you are at a business breakfast or coffee, and one muffin remains on the tray in the middle of the table. Do you feel you are the only person who is secretly worried about what is going to become of that muffin?

One way to deal with the tremendous number of choices that your mind must make on any given day is to establish behaviors with livable but definable borders. Actually, many good food choices can be made on business trips and in airports. Review the list below, and see which ones will fit in with your game plan.

Travel Eating Tips

1. *Alter your eating routine as little as possible.* If you go on a two-week vacation and eat everything in sight, it could take you another six months to regain control. Or dieting for a week while at home and then letting yourself go for a week while traveling will result in

a net of nothing—if you're lucky. Attempt to eat foods and portions that are your normal routine.

2. *Take along special diet aids,* such as low-cal salad dressing packets and butter sprinkles. These can even come in handy on airplanes.

3. *Take opportunities to walk and exercise* wherever you may be. Airport terminals are great places to stretch your legs. Just pretend that you are walking fast to catch a plane. You'll look like everyone else. And many hotels now have exercise facilities. So take advantage! You can even look for hotels that have adjoining shopping malls that can serve as a safe walking track.

4. *Take along a concrete reminder* that you are living with a new set of rules. For example, in your daytimer add a section that is a food journal. Every time you eat or drink anything at all, write it down. It doesn't have to be perfect, but at least make it honest. A small, spiral notebook stuck in your pocket can serve the same purpose. When you are tempted to reach for the four-inch brownie in Atlanta, remember that you have to write it down in your diary.

5. *Enlist the aid of a friend* if all else fails, and be accountable for your pre- and post-trip weight to this person. If you belong to a weight-loss group in your area, make a point to attend after you return from the trip instead of skipping that week.

6. *Nurture yourself in other ways* with a new dress, manicure, jogging suit, or even a fashion magazine. Learn to be a connoisseur of good coffees, teas, and other non-caloric beverages.

7. *Make a point to drink fluids,* which may not be as readily available while you are traveling. Fast-food places are happy to refill your own thermos and cups with ice water. Squeeze in a packet or wedge of lemon for a fresh taste in your water. Airplanes are notorious for their dry atmosphere and can dehydrate you.

8. *Don't be swayed by an expense account.* You are only hurting yourself when you eat to enjoy your expense account or "get what's coming to you." Think of how many dollars you have spent on weight loss. Does it now seem sensible to consume more than you want so that you can get your share? Your company will even appreciate a more controlled palate, which uses less of its resources.

How to Find a Lowfat Meal in the Air

You've made your reservations, booked the hotel, your intentions are good, and the food diary is in your pocket. Now the time has come to actually follow through. The good news is that airlines are increasingly attempting to meet consumer demands for more nutritious, lowfat fare. All major airlines now offer a wide variety of special meals, ranging from kosher to gluten-free. By giving the airline reservation desk (or your travel agent) only twenty-four hours notice, you can have one of these special menus on your next flight.

If you are looking for a lowfat meal with adequate fruits and vegetables, try the lowfat, low-cholesterol fruit plate, or the vegetarian or cold seafood plate. The *low-cholesterol meal* usually includes skinless, boneless chicken; vegetables; tossed salad; bread; light dressing; and fresh fruit. The lowfat plate is usually similar. With *the cold seafood plate,* the salad itself will be a high-protein, lowfat choice. The accompanying dressings and desserts may not be. *Fruit plates* can be a good choice if a high-fat cheese is not included. Fruit and cottage cheese is great, whereas a brick cheese and croissant would dismantle all your good intentions. Likewise, for the *vegetarian plate,* high-fat sources of protein are often included, such as cheese and/or peanut butter.

The best choice for nutritious airline food is the lowfat or low-cholesterol plate. I usually find that they are also better quality food. Many passengers look at these entrées and wish they had thought to make this request. The following chart further summarizes the choices that are available to you.

Special Airline Meals

	American	British Airways	Continental	Delta	Eastern	Lufthansa	Midway	Northwest	Pan Am	TWA	USAir	United
Hours required prior to departure	12	24	12	8	8	24	24	8	8	24	24	24
Religious												
Kosher	•	•	•	•	•	•	•	•	•	•	•	•
Hindu	•	•	•	•	•	•			•	•		•
Muslim	•	•	•	•	•	•		•	•			•
Medical												
Bland	•	•		•	•	•		•	•			•
Diabetic/Low sugar	•	•	•	•	•	•		•	•	•	•	•
Gluten-free		•		•	•			•	•			•
Low-calorie	•	•		•	•	•		•	•	•	•	•
Low-carbohydrate	•	•		•	•			•		•		•
Low-cholesterol	•	•	•	•	•	•		•				•
Lowfat	•				•				•	•	•	
Low-sodium	•	•	•	•	•	•		•	•	•	•	•
Other												
Fruit Plate	•			•	•			•	•		•	•
Seafood, Hot				•				•	•			
Seafood, Cold	•			•	•	•		•	•	•		•
Infant		•	•	•				•				•
Toddler				•	•							
Child	•	•	•	•	•		•	•	•	•	•	•
Vegetarian, strict		•	•	•	•			•				
Vegetarian, ovo/lacto	•	•	•	•	•	•	•	•	•	•	•	•

Reprinted with permission from Environmental Nutrition Newsletter, 2112 Broadway, Ste. 200, New York, NY 10023.

It is wise to confirm your special meal twenty-four hours prior to departure. If you use the same travel agency on all of your bookings, they can keep this information in your travel profile and order these automatically with each ticket. In case of a last-minute change in flight plan, don't expect your special meal (or your bags!) to make the flight. But try to keep your cool. Don't fall for the extra butter, salad dressing, and heavy dessert presented on the regular meal and think you can still come out okay.

If you anticipate layovers during mealtimes, pack something in your briefcase. A 110-calorie banana can go a long way in curbing a rising appetite. And, just maybe, it can keep you from succumbing to that 500-calorie brownie in Atlanta!

PARTY HARDY, BUT DON'T DITCH THE DIET

There is no problem with that once or twice a year Turkey Day binge. We're Americans; you expect that kind of thing. When this type of simple tradition takes on recreational status, however, you can bet that weight gain is sure to follow.

Here are some tips on behaviors, snack alternatives, and healthy foods to serve at parties.

Party-Perfect Habits

First, decide approximately how many calories you should consume at the get-together. You may skip one meal (such as the evening meal if it is a nighttime party), but do not fast all day in preparation or go hungry to the party, because you may eat everything in sight when you get there.

Second, instead of picking up bits of this and that, fix yourself a plate of food that meets your calorie requirements for the day. Then avoid returning to the buffet table.

Third, try to avoid alcoholic and other caloric beverages because they add up fast. Alcohol is actually more calorically concentrated than rice, potatoes, or sugar. Choose sparkling mineral water with a twist of lime or lemon. Diet sodas are also an option.

Fourth, when choosing foods, attempt to place a large selection of fruits, vegetables (easy on the dip, though), sandwiches, low-cal crackers, and lean meats on your plate. These will help fill your stomach for fewer calories than sweets, potato chips, and dips.

Fifth, the worst selections on any party table are those items made from cream cheese, sour cream, mayonnaise, cheese, cheese dips, chips, nuts, fatty meats, and butter. Also be careful with baked sweets. Most of these contain from 50 to 95 percent fat.

Sixth, do a lot of talking at the party. It will keep your mind off food. Make a point to speak to at least five people.

Seventh, exercise at some point during the day before your party to help cut your appetite, give you more energy and vitality, and help you feel good about your new choices.

And last, wear something nice-looking to nurture your feelings of self-confidence.

Prime Party Fare You Can Make

- Try some new and unusual vegetables in your vegetable dips, such as jicama. Trust me on this one. It looks like a big, ugly turnip but has a pleasing crunch and almost a sweet taste. To serve as a vegetable dipper, simply peel and cut into long strips as you might make carrot sticks. Also try raw zucchini, yellow squash, and radish coins as vegetable dippers. Use an ordinary straw basket, lined on the inside with ruffly lettuce leaves, and then stuff cut-up vegetable sticks in as if they were in an ornamental flower arrangement. It makes a great centerpiece.

- Make vegetable dips out of puréed cottage cheese (use a food processor) and any spice package or combination you like. Ranch party dip is especially nice for this. Add a tablespoon of lemon juice for a sour cream taste. The recipe for this dip is on page 227.

- Use the vegetable dip described above to spread over pita bread or, better yet, eight-inch tortillas. When using tortillas, spread it over the entire surface area, roll the tortilla, and then cut into thirds so that each piece is about two inches long. The tortillas will stick together with this dip on the inside and look like a pinwheel. Arrange on a platter, and serve with a bowl of picante sauce in the middle.

- Fruit is best served at a finger-food party when skewered. It can be easily handled in this way and is not messy for your party guests. Choose fruits that will not get soft or turn brown after sitting out awhile, such as apples, pears, or bananas. Strawberries, mandarin oranges, and grapes are better choices for this serving method. You can use standard toothpicks or the small bamboo skewers available at many party warehouses.

- Snack-sized beef, chicken, or shrimp shish-kebabs can be made on small skewers. You can use bite-sized pieces of meat with cherry tomatoes and other vegetables marinated for tenderness, including bell pepper and pearl onions. If you have an indoor grill, cook this while your guests wait and watch with anticipation. Serve as they come off the grill.

- Begin with an inexpensive frozen cheese pizza. Add some imported Romano and Parmesan cheeses (the very pungent varieties) and top with very thinly sliced bell pepper, onion, mushroom, and zucchini slices. Cut into 2-inch squares and arrange on a tray.

- Finger sandwiches are always a hit at parties when people have come from work and want "real food," not just junk. You can make lowfat tuna, chicken, or crab meat spreads using light Miracle Whip by Kraft and finely chopped vegetables (celery, onion, pickle, cucumber) as additional fillers. Use light breads if everyone is dieting. If you use all light products, a finger sandwich might be only fifty calories, depending on the thickness of the spread.

- Using a food processor to make dips and sandwich spreads allows them to be very spreadable and well blended.

- Rice cakes make a wonderful base for decorated canapes. Don't make them too early in the day or they will get soggy.

- Make use of the lighter varieties of chips and lowfat crackers. Remember that picante sauce has virtually no calories and makes an excellent dip. Tostado chips now come in a lowfat, baked variety from the company called Guiltless Gourmet®. Ask your grocer for this brand by name. They have great products.

BENEFIT FROM GOOD BEHAVIORS

Behavior modification has been rehashed in many diet books, ours included. To be complete, it is necessary to say a few words about this important area, even if you have heard these words before. I want to first discuss the American eating style. Think about your own life as I discuss this issue, and get really honest about how you live.

When I was in graduate school getting a Ph.D. in nutrition, I rarely found time to eat nutritiously or with a spirit of calmness. In fact, most of my lunches came from an antiquated (but fully functional) snack machine that was actually in the nutrition building. The cafeteria was across campus, and in those days, I wasn't much on exercise. I hardly ever had the foresight to bring my lunch; so if I was going to eat, it was likely to be out of this machine. Sometimes I visited this machine more than once. It was quick, easy, and I could rationalize that I was eating crackers. Do you know that most of the chocolate bars in that machine had less fat in them than the cheese crackers I chose for lunch most days?

Other meals were usually eaten in my car. I had a thirty-minute commute to school and was not organized enough to settle into a routine of breakfast before I left. And in all honesty, I think I nurtured myself with food in the car.

There are several problems with this type of lifestyle, and I have talked to enough of my patients to know that many of you are living like this right now. First, if you are constantly on the run, you may be rewarding yourself with food for never having time to yourself. Flee from this lifestyle scenario, and do whatever is necessary to get out of that breakneck fast lane. Next, food eaten while on the run sometimes "doesn't count" in your mind. You may think that the three-hundred-calorie package of crackers and peanut butter were so small that they just don't matter. Isn't that what you are tempted to think at times?

Snacking on anything in any place is simply not good training for your new lifestyle. From previous *Love Hunger* books, you learned that you don't need food as an emotional crutch anymore. You can get through that workday without giving yourself an edible perk. You don't have to run for chocolate because you can't stand your boss. You are a new person now, concerned with healthy decision making.

Experts agree that "appropriate eating areas" must be chosen for your meals. It requires that you establish mealtimes and stick to them. It does not mean that you eat when you are not hungry. But, it does mean that you spread your food throughout the entire day and take time and care in preparing your food and nurturing yourself in this healthy way.

Ideally, you should eat at a table with a full set of dishes and in a pleasant atmosphere. You can eat alone or with others. You should not watch television while you eat or consistently be engaged in another activity in tandem with mealtime. Avoid eating at your desk at work. Avoid eating in your car. Avoid eating on your couch or bed. Eat to feed yourself, not for entertainment.

Additionally, get used to drinking a lot of fluids. You may keep a drink handy on your desk or while you watch television. Try water with lemon, mineral water, spring water, diet sodas, and other sugar-free drinks. Coffee and tea are okay too. If you are really hungry, try a bouillon cube in hot water. It will help cut your appetite until mealtime.

I won't ask you to chew each bite thirty times (yuck!), but I do want you to slow down your rate of eating. Eating should be done slowly, savoring each bite, knowing that you will not go back for seconds. Lay down your fork to get a drink of water. These kinds of things are important because of the *twenty-minute rule*. It takes twenty minutes for the food you have just eaten to reach your stomach, be partially digested, get into your bloodstream, and into your brain to turn off the hunger center. Have you ever eaten a very large meal, thought you were still hungry, but felt overstuffed? It is possible to feel overfull and still be somewhat hungry. Guard against this by taking your time when eating or by having a low-cal appetizer before the meal begins (soup or salad).

Let's go on to the next section, now, and discover ways to work off calories and deplete fat cells through a complete fitness program.

Enjoy Fitness as Part of Your New Lifestyle

Exercise should be your greatest dieting, weight-loss, and weight-maintenance ally. Though some of us (me included) once pegged it as the *E* word and thought it was the albatross that wouldn't go home, anyone can change course by 180 degrees. Whereas I once struggled to make it around the block and back, I now thrive on a five-mile walk/run. It is actually great fun and a private time for me.

As you are deciding if you are really going to make increased activity part of your new and healthier lifestyle, consider these facts:

- Exercise can increase your rate of weight loss by up to one-third or even half. That is, if you were going to lose two pounds for the week by diet alone, you might lose three pounds by including exercise.
- Exercise can help build calorie-burning muscles. Even at rest, muscles burn eight times more calories than an equal amount of fat. Thus, building muscles can help you maintain your weight loss even while you sleep!

- Exercise improves your attitude and outlook on life through endorphin stimulation. It is a main line of treatment for mild depression, anxiety, and stress reduction.
- Exercise makes you look good and feel better.
- Exercise helps motivate people who have unsuccessfully dieted in the past.
- Exercise improves muscle tone and conditioning, and makes you feel more energetic.
- Exercise improves your immune system so that your body's own natural defenses against illness and disease are enhanced.
- Exercise decreases your chances of developing cardiovascular disease, diabetes, high blood pressure, and elevated levels of blood cholesterol and triglycerides.
- Exercise can often improve premenstrual syndrome symptoms.
- Exercising one hour per day usually means you can sleep one hour less because you sleep more efficiently and effectively.

It is usually not difficult to convince someone that they need to be more active. The difficult part enters in when they attempt to change what has become a habitually sedative lifestyle.

Let's face it. Humans (especially those past the age of thirty-something) hate change. We get set in our ways. We think, "Why change, now?" OK—here it comes. I'm only going to say it once. Most experts agree that if obese dieters do not make an equal commitment to exercise consistently along with dieting, they will never enjoy dieting success and weight maintenance. Flatly, you can't get weight off and keep it off without a fitness program of your own.

Part of this mega-pronouncement has to do with maintenance. If you make a commitment to walk thirty minutes per day (roughly two miles or an expenditure of 200 calories) for five days per week, this could keep you from gaining about fifteen pounds in a one year's period of time.

If you have the genetic predisposition for weight gain, you must consider ways of changing what has commonly been called your "setpoint," or the weight that your genes tell you to weigh. Burning an extra 800 to 2000 calories per week is no doubt part of a package that will help keep you in control.

If you are wavering on beginning your own exercise program, consider these facts:

- Exercise requires very little in the way of equipment. Good shoes and loose, cool clothes are the only "must haves."

- You do not have to join a health club or spa to be fit. See the workout program on the following pages, for example.

- Be gentle with yourself and progress in stages.

- You can start today. Make time for this. It needs to be at the top of your priority list.

- It takes no more than a two-hour-per-week commitment to greatly improve your cardiovascular fitness. That's the time it takes to watch one video rental.

MAKING THE MOST OF AEROBICS

Aerobics is the key element of an effective weight-loss exercise program. Aerobic simply means that your heart (which is a muscle) is being exercised at 65 to 80 percent of its maximum potential. When this happens you are not only doing your cardiovascular system a big favor, but you are also mobilizing your metabolism into action. Exercise is a sure cure for anyone with a sluggish metabolism and overall lethargy. It may sound a little crazy to advise exercise for those who are tired, but documented studies show that this is just what works.

As you exercise aerobically, your heart rate increases its pace. This is how you actually determine if you are engaged in an aerobic activity. Find your target heart-rate range below:

Target Heart-Rate Range

Age	Safe Range/Min. (beats/min.)	Maximum (beats/min.)
20	140–170	200
30	130–162	190
40	126–158	180
50	119–145	170
60	112–136	160
70	105–128	150

The key elements about aerobic exercise to remember are these:

Duration   You must maintain the exercise for a minimum of 20 minutes.

Intensity   You should be between 65 and 85 percent of your maximum heart rate.

Steadiness   The exercise must be nonstop and consistent.

Frequency   You need to exercise

- six days per week to improve fitness and help lose weight.
- four days per week to maintain fitness and weight.
- two days a week or less means that your level of fitness will decline.

TYPES OF AEROBIC ACTIVITIES

Walking Is Still Number One

Nothing could be easier or more pleasant than putting on a comfortable pair of shoes and leaving all your cares behind while you make a quick getaway through a park or even down your street. Enjoy the birds, the sights, the sounds, or even a novel on tape while you walk. Much has already been written on regular walking, so in this section I want to give special discussion to that weird-looking, hip-swivelling race walker that passes you by somedays and makes you look like you're standing still. First, we just have to get by the impulse to laugh at them, just as we snickered at joggers only 15 years ago. Walking isn't merely locomotion, but an activity with several potential variations, including walking at the Olympic level. In 1983, the world record for a mile walk was set by American Ray Sharp: 5 minutes, 46 seconds. That's phenomenal! I can't run a mile in that length of time! Most of us plod along at about a mile in fifteen minutes and are elated with that.

We can't all be Olympians, but racewalking offers many benefits to the walker who has gotten into good shape and is now ready for a new challenge. Racewalking can burn as many calories per hour as running, but with much less risk of injury. It's not an expensive sport and requires nothing save decent walking clothing and shoes.

The Finer Points of Racewalking

The object of racewalking is to move your body ahead as quickly as possible (without running) and to avoid the up/down motions of regular walking. That is the point of the forward-thrusting hip-swivel, which is meant to propel you more efficiently than the normal side-to-side swing of the hips. Now, here's how to start:

1. Think of racewalking as walking a tightrope. In normal walking, you will make parallel tracks; but in racewalking you must try to put one foot down in front of the other, as if you are walking on an imaginary straight line. Because of anatomical variations, this form may not be possible for everyone, but try to come as close to this as possible.

2. Swing your hip forward as you step forward. The hips propel you.

3. Keep your feet close to the ground with no wasted motion or effort. Each foot should strike the ground on the back of the heel with

the toes pointed slightly upward. A competition rule of racewalking is that one foot must always be on the ground.

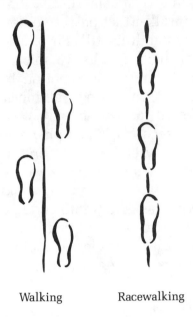

Walking   Racewalking

4. Use long strides. Your motion should be a fluid movement and should feel efficient and smooth.

5. Keep your torso, neck, and shoulders relaxed and your head in line with your back. Don't bend from the waist, since this can lead to back strain. Some racewalkers angle their whole body slightly forward from the ankles.

6. Bend your arms at a 90-degree angle, and keep your wrists straight. With the motions coming from the shoulder, not the elbow, pump your arms rhythmically in sync with your legs. When your arm pumps backward, your hand should come about six inches behind the hip; while on the swing forward, the wrist should come near the center of the chest. Keep your hands above your hips as they swing. This vigorous hand and arm motion counterbalances the leg movements and helps propel you at a faster pace. It also provides a good workout for the upper body (a badly neglected area).

7. Experience is necessary to do well with racewalking. Contact someone in your area to help you with the finer points.

8. If this seems too difficult at first, try interval walking—where you walk briskly (but not racewalk), switch to racewalking, and then slow down again. Be patient with yourself and make it enjoyable.

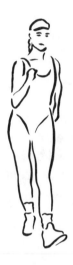

Try Sprouting Some Fins

Swimming can be the best aerobic exercise, particularly when you have joint problems, arthritis, or some type of injury that precludes load-bearing exercise. Swimming can help you burn up to three hundred calories per thirty-minute session and exercises all of the major muscle groups. But many swimmers find the freestyle technique or stroke difficult and end up struggling to keep their bodies properly aligned. Here are some tips that may be helpful:

1. When you are taking a slow freestyle pace, make sure you exhale completely before you turn your head to the side for another breath. Otherwise you will be breathing more than you need to. Don't hold your head high in the water when breathing. In fact, the water level should just be at your hairline. To inhale, turn your head just far enough to the side to breathe. Catch a breath every two or three strokes.

2. Kick from the hips, not the knees. Use your thigh and buttock muscles to do this. To maintain a streamlined form in the water, keep your feet close to the surface. In fact, the heel of the kicking foot should break the surface of the water, and the other foot should be no more than one foot deep. Some trainers suggest kicking two or three times per stroke, but you need to set your own pace.

3. Don't push water straight back. Instead, use your hands to trace an "S" pattern through the water. This will help propel you at a faster speed and more efficiently. In short, it will make this activity more fun!

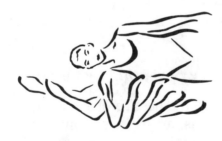

4. It never hurts to ask a qualified swimming instructor to give you a refresher course. Adult lessons are usually available at the local YMCA for a reasonable fee.

5. If you are uncertain about your swimming abilities or have never really felt comfortable with the freestyle stroke, you may use a small styrofoam "boogie board" that supports your arms and keeps your head above water. Then you merely kick your feet as we have described, and you are off! You don't even have to be a good swimmer for this activity. (Stick to a swimming pool rather than a lake or ocean if you can't swim well.)

Step up to Fitness

Do you remember high school coaches who would make you run the stairs at the bleachers when training suddenly became "serious"? Maybe they had something. Climbing stairs is actually a great way to get in shape, have a cardiovascular workout, and lose weight. To do this, though, you have to use an exercise video with a portable step, live in an area that has many stairs to climb, or use a stair stepper machine.

Consumer Reports (May 1992) says there are no less-expensive home versions that can really compete with the commercial stair steppers found at fitness clubs. Still, they found some that were better than others. Check their magazine for brand names. Now here are some tips that will help you get the most out of your stair stepping:

- Avoid leaning into the handrails except for balance only. If you lean on them to reduce your weight, then you also reduce the load on your legs.

- To prevent knee strain, keep knees directly over toes.

- Increase your time first, then add speed and difficulty. Start with short steps. Once you have had plenty of experience with the machine, increase your step depth and speed. Keep your workouts challenging.

- Use distractions to fight boredom. Watching television or listening to music (or a novel on tape) is a great use of your time.

Bench Aerobics

Another version of stair steppers is the single step or bench, which is being used in aerobic classes and on exercise videos throughout the country. This small platform (often made of molded plastic) is about the height of one stair step. Working to music, you step on and off the bench in a routine that gives you a cardiovascular workout while it tones legs and buttocks. And it's low impact, since one foot is always on the floor or on the step.

Have you ever tried one of these "Step Classes" at the local YMCA or health club? They are really tough. Essentially, it is a challenging, fast-paced way to do low-impact aerobics. Two recent studies from San Diego State University looked at specific benefits from step training. One of them found that a rate of 120 steps per minute while pumping the arms required the same exertion as running a seven-minute mile. Yet the impact was equivalent to only walking at three miles per hour. In a University of Pittsburgh study, subjects working at eighty steps per minute burned almost three hundred calories in thirty minutes. The calorie expenditure increased 19 percent when one-pound hand weights and a pumping arm motion were added.

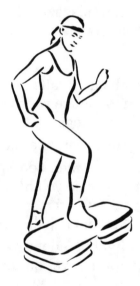

Step aerobic classes are popping up all over the place. There is probably one available in your area. I personally enjoy doing this activity with a group, since I feel that I push myself harder to keep up with everyone else. But, as is true for any fitness program, you need to start slow. Beginners should use a four-inch step, increasing the height eventually to eight and even twelve inches. If you plan to purchase a bench and work out at home, take a few classes to learn the necessary coordination and technique. Always place your sole (not your toes or the ball of your foot) flat on the center of the platform, keep your knee slightly bent. Land back on the floor with the ball of your foot, then bring your heel down smoothly, bending your knee as you do so to absorb the impact. You may have to look down at your feet when you're just starting.

The regular stepping will be enough of a challenge in the beginning stages. After you feel comfortable with this, add hand weights and pump your arms as you step. One- to three-pound hand or wrist weights will be the correct choice. As with any exercise program, press yourself to fatigue just a little with each workout. Eventually, you will be able to do more, assuming you are exercising at least four times per week.

Commercially available benches, made of high-impact plastic or wood, are about forty-two inches long and fourteen inches wide with adjustable height and nonskid surfaces. Plastic ones don't have any sharp corners or splinters—they are my personal favorites. *Do not* try this with a regular household footstool.

Take the Laid-back Approach with Recumbent Biking

Recumbent biking has actually been around since the early 1800s. In the last few years, however, stationary models are seen in many health spas with greater frequency. These bikes are lower to the ground and longer than regular stationary bikes. You sit in an upright position in an oversized seat with a back support while your legs stretch out horizontally to do the peddling. It is quite comfortable—almost like riding an old kiddie-car type toy. Advantages of recumbent biking include:

- greater back support and general comfort;
- a different type of workout for your muscles: the muscles of the buttocks and hamstrings are worked to a greater degree than standard cycling; and
- a good aerobic workout particularly suited for those who are not fit; your blood pressure may not rise as much as during upright cycling because your legs are nearly at the level of your heart.

Get a Jump on Fitness

How long has it been since you've tried "hot peppers" with a skipping rope? Believe it or not, jumping rope is on the upswing. You can pack a jump rope in a suitcase, do it on rainy days, and it certainly doesn't require a lot of elaborate equipment. Let's look at some of the aerobic, weight loss, and fitness benefits of jumping rope.

- Jumping rope helps build endurance, just like cycling, swimming, and jogging. It is just as strenuous as jogging and provides a good cardiovascular workout.
- Jumping rope is a good calorie burner. If you weigh 150 pounds and jump at a beginner's rate of seventy skips per minute, you'll burn eleven calories per minute. This is the same as running at a pace of about six miles per hour.
- Jumping rope is a lower impact exercise than jogging, since your goal is to jump no more than one inch off the ground.
- It is an alternative exercise for those accustomed to outdoor exercise.

To get started, begin with a slow pace of about seventy skips per minute. There are two basic ways to jump: on one foot at a time, alternating feet as in a jogging motion. Or on two feet at a time at a little quicker pace. You may vary your routine by swinging the rope forward or backward or by being stationary or moving around. Try watching the evening news while you skip rope. You will expend 220 calories in only twenty minutes.

It is best to jump rope one to three times per week—not every day so that you don't overdo a good thing by putting too much continual pressure on your joints. You will need a good pair of supportive shoes (the same ones you use for walking or jogging) and a rope to get started. Make sure the rope handles fit comfortably in your hands and that the rope turns easily where it is connected to the handles. The kind with a ball-bearing construction is a good choice. You can find these at sporting goods stores, usually for less than ten dollars. To check the rope length, stand on the center of the rope and pull the handles up the sides of your body. They should just come up to your armpits. Some ropes come with instructions for adjusting the length. Wooden floors are the best jumping surface, but almost anything works as long as the rope and shoes are good.

Find Balance, Fitness, and Weight Loss with Circuit Training

Circuit training is the combination of aerobic exercise interspersed with weight training. Weight training is a hybrid between weight lifting with small weights and calisthenics. It is a balanced approach to fitness that gives you an effective cardiovascular workout as well as some high-intensity exercise for increasing muscle strength. This is the type of exercise we call *toning*. It strengthens and increases the size of your muscles lying underneath the subcutaneous layer of fat that surrounds them. Thus, circuit training helps with weight loss and cellulite control.

Like an electrical circuit with energy popping along a defined pathway, circuit training may be thought of in similar fashion. After a brief warm-up, you will begin with a twenty-minute aerobic workout of your choice. It could be a brisk walk around your neighborhood, stationary biking, or any of the other aerobic activities listed above. Time yourself and return to your workout area after twenty minutes.

Next you will alternate between a set of exercises and more short aerobic sessions. The exercises often make use of small hand-held weights (two-, three-, or five- pound weights) and leg weights (one or two pound). These should be in your exercise area and readily accessible before you begin the exercise session. Using these weights will add extra resistance to your muscles and help build lean body mass.

The purpose of the short aerobic spurts midway in the exercises is to keep you at an aerobic pace for the duration of the exercise session. Keep in mind that after the first thirty to forty minutes of rather intense exercise you start burning almost pure fat as a fuel source. To keep your heart at an aerobic pace during the floor exercises, do not take long breaks between sets or stop for other reasons. (Take the phone off the hook!) Ultimately, you will lose body fat, improve your muscle tone, increase your cardiovascular fitness, and improve cellulite areas. Try to repeat this program four or five times per week with extra walking as desired.

The following pages will provide you with all the information you need to do your own at-home circuit training. Gradually build up to the suggested number of repetitions. When you are able to do the entire program, it should take about forty-five minutes to one hour. This program will be too difficult for some of you to begin at the top level of repetitions. *Please* be kind to yourself and try to reach small goals each week. If you strain yourself in the beginning, you might be unable to work out for weeks. You have plenty of time to reach those goals. Remember, you have made a commitment to do this for the rest of your life.

AT-HOME CIRCUIT TRAINING PROGRAM

Basic instructions:

1. Wear comfortable clothing suited to your aerobic choice.

2. Have small barbells (start with two pounds and progress to five) readily available. Likewise, have the leg weights (one or two pound) close so that they may be put on quickly.

3. Go quickly from one exercise to the other. Keep up your pace so that your heart rate will stay at aerobic pace for the duration of the workout.

4. Attempt to eliminate distractions, such as the telephone. Ask children to entertain themselves for this brief period of time. Or exercise during naptime if you have small children. Television watching is okay if you can still adequately concentrate on your weight training. I personally prefer music.

5. If you will be jogging or walking, make sure you have supportive shoes meant for this purpose.

Warm-Ups

The following five exercises form the warm-up section. It is *very important* that you complete this section before each exercise session. This is especially true when your body is cold. Pulling one muscle can put you out of commission for up to three weeks. Don't risk it by skipping your warm-ups.

Neck Stretch

Stand tall with good posture and legs apart. Slowly rotate your head to the right, stopping when your ear is over your shoulder. Then, rotate to the left. Slowly, gently, stretch your neck as far as you can four times on each side. Now slowly roll your head in circles toward the right four times and then toward the left four times.

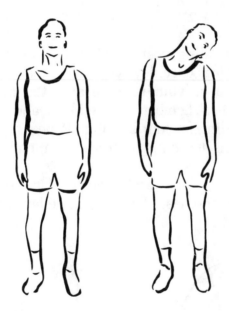

Shoulder Shrug

Continue standing with straight posture. Now raise your shoulders as high as possible and hold for three seconds as you breathe deeply. Roll your shoulders back down and breathe out. Repeat for a total of eight times.

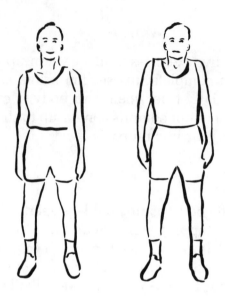

Back Stretch

From your standing position slowly bend over and run your hands down your legs to achieve your own greatest stretch. Attempt to touch the floor as you improve over the next few months. Straighten both legs. Then bend the left knee and stretch down over the right leg, holding for four seconds. Repeat the stretch over the left leg. Repeat this stretching exercise for a total of eight times on each side.

Bend both knees and straighten to a standing position very slowly. Keep arms and head dangling and relaxed until you reach a standing position.

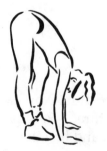 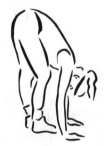

Leg Stretch Number 1

Stand facing a wall. Place your hands on the wall in front of you. Put the left leg near the wall in a bent position and extend the right leg back. Slowly lower your right heel to the floor and hold for a count of four. Feel the stretch in the back of your right leg. Release the right leg and repeat this exercise seven more times.

Exchange leg positions and stretch the left leg eight times.

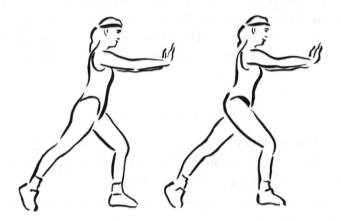

Leg Stretch Number 2

Stand facing a wall. Place your left hand on the wall with arm slightly bent. Stand on your left leg. Raise the right leg so that the right hand can grasp the right ankle from the back as shown below. Pull on the right ankle as you feel the stretch. Hold in the stretched position for a count of ten. Repeat with your left leg for a count of ten.

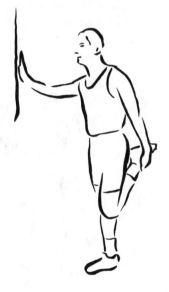

Aerobics—Twenty Minutes

You are now warmed up, and it should be safe for you to exert your muscles further. Choose any of the aerobics listed previously (walking, jogging, recumbent or stationary biking, outdoor biking, jump roping, or swimming), and continue the chosen activity for twenty minutes.

Hint: To help yourself flow more smoothly from aerobics to calisthenics, have on your exercise gear prior to warm-ups. That way you could warm up in your living room, walk right out your front door for a twenty-minute walk, and then return for the next set of exercises.

Upper Torso Exercises

All of the following exercises will use small, hand-held weights, from one to ten pounds. These pieces of equipment should be in the room before you begin your workout.

Arm Raises with Weights

Pick up your small barbells and hold one in each hand. Stand with feet apart, legs straight, and toes slightly turned out. Hold bar-

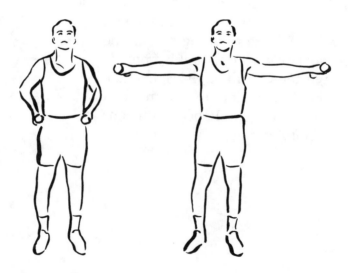

bells with arms bent and hands at hips. Raise barbells to about shoulder level, keeping arms slightly bent; and then lower fairly slowly. Repeat for a total of twelve lifts. Shake arms for a few seconds, and then repeat for another set of twelve lifts.

Forearm Lifts

Stand with legs apart. Hold barbells with hands cupped toward the front of the body. Bring hands to the chest. Repeat for a total of twelve lifts. Take a few seconds to shake out your arms, and then repeat this exercise for two more sets of twelve. (Do three sets for a total of 36 lifts.)

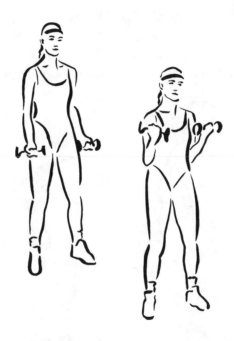

Arm Extensions

Bend over at hips with barbells in hands. Keep your legs and back straight. With barbells, let your arms hang loose. Raise the barbells to your chest with elbows extended outward. Repeat for a total of thirty times. Rest halfway through if you need to for two sets of fifteen.

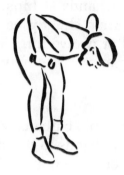

Rear Arm Extensions

Stand with legs apart at shoulder width and knees bent. Hold barbells at about hip level with arms slightly bent. Raise the arms backwards as far as possible. Repeat for a total of twelve times. Rest a few seconds, and repeat for two more sets of twelve.

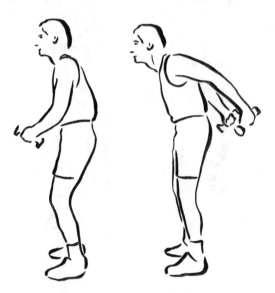

Seated Arm Raises

Sit in a chair with your legs together; keep your back straight; and place your left hand on your hip. (As an option you may perform this exercise in the standing position.) With a barbell in your right hand, drop your hand over the back of your right shoulder and then lift straight up as far as you can reach. Feel the stretch in the back of your arm. Repeat for a total of twelve times. Then switch to the left arm. Rest for a few seconds and then repeat twelve more on each arm.

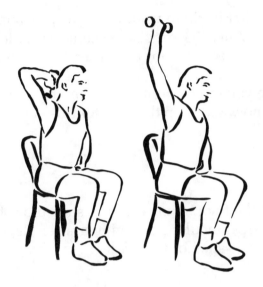

Modified Push-ups

Begin on hands and knees. Keep your back straight. Bend arms to lower your head and chest as close to the floor as possible. Do not let your back either crest or sag. Repeat for a total of twelve. Rest a few seconds and do one more set of twelve.

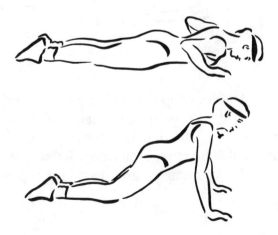

Aerobics—Six Minutes

Leg Exercises

When you first begin to work with this program, you need not use leg weights. After the exercises become easier for you, use one- to three-pound leg weights for each exercise as shown in the pictures.

It will take you only a minute to sit on the floor and put on the weights. Do it now and keep them on for this entire section of exercises.

Leg Lifts

Lie flat on the floor. Arms and legs should be straight. Lift the right leg to a perpendicular position or greater. Repeat for a total of thirty lifts. Do the same for the left leg.

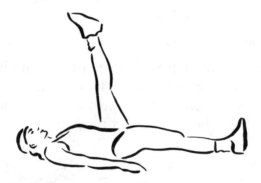

Side Leg Lifts

Lie on your left side. Keep the left leg straight and bend the right leg, placing the right foot behind the left leg. Support the upper torso with the left arm. Put the right forearm in front of the body with the hand on the floor (see picture). Raise and lower the left leg for a total of thirty times. Turn over and repeat on the other side.

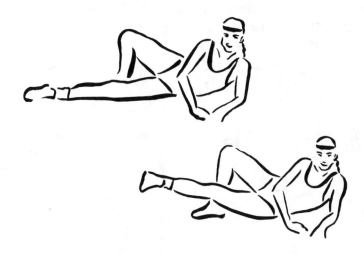

Rear Leg Lifts

Lie facedown on the floor with legs together and arms straight by the side. Lift the right leg toward the ceiling as far as possible, keeping the leg straight. Now lift the left leg. Repeat this series for a total of thirty times on each leg.

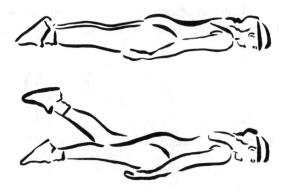

Leg Extensions and Contractions

Begin on hands and knees. Lower your head and bring the left leg into your chest. Then, raise head, extend the left leg backward and upward. Repeat by bringing the left leg into the chest and lowering your chin to meet your knee. Repeat this in-and-out motion for a total count of twenty. Do the same with the right leg.

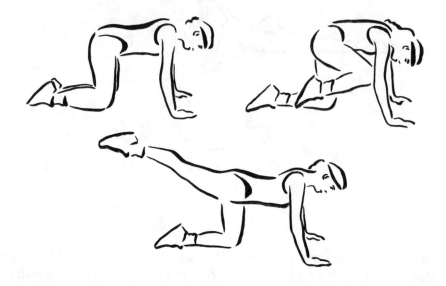

Backward Leg Lifts

Begin on all fours, and then extend your left leg with toe touching floor. Now lift the left leg straight up, keeping it straight, and lower. Repeat twenty times; then do the same on the other leg.

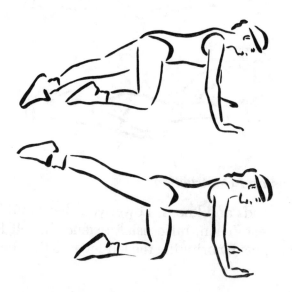

Leg Swings

Hold onto a chair or bar with the right hand. Stand erect. Raise the left leg forward, then raise to the back. Reverse the exercise and swing the right leg. Repeat for a total of twenty swings on each leg.

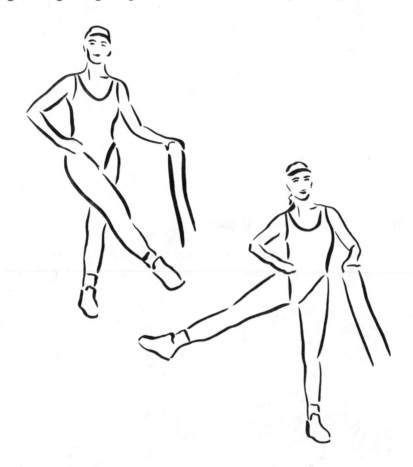

Twisting Exercise

With slightly bent knees, stand tall with your feet apart. Extend your arms straight out at shoulder height. Keep the lower part of your body stationary, and twist from side to side in helicopter fashion. Repeat for a total of fifty twists, alternating to the right and to the left.

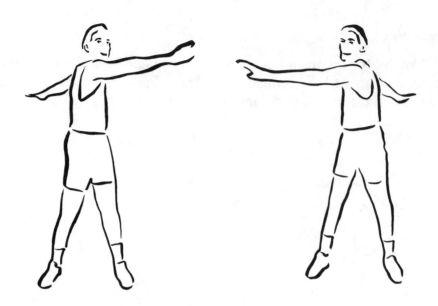

Forward Leg Lifts Using Weights

Sit in a tall chair with your back straight. With a barbell held between your feet, raise and lower your legs. Repeat for a total of thirty times.

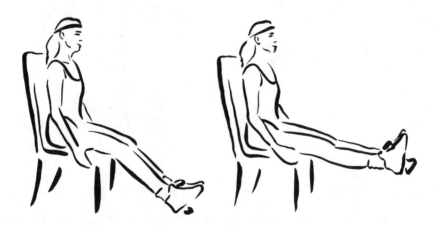

Backward Leg Lifts Using Weights

(Optional exercise depending on whether or not you have an appropriate area.)

Find a nearby step area similar to the picture shown below. Lie down and support your upper torso on your forearms. Holding a barbell between your feet, raise and lower your legs, bending at the knee. Repeat thirty times.

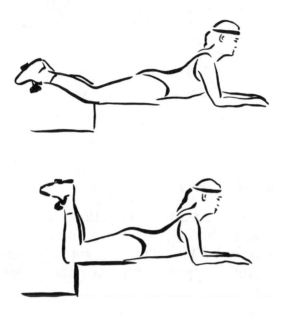

Aerobics

Do your aerobics for seven more minutes. You may take off your leg weights at this point.

Stomach Exercises

Stomach Crunch Number 1

Begin with your head on the floor, hands clasped behind the head and knees bent. Raise your head and upper torso as far as possible, keeping your lower back and hips on the floor. Point your elbows toward your knees as you pull yourself up. Repeat twenty times.

Rest for five seconds, and repeat twenty more crunches—except that your elbows should point toward the ceiling as you raise yourself.

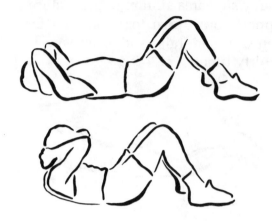

Stomach Crunch Number 2

From your current position on the floor, reach toward your left knee with your right elbow and attempt to touch them together. Now switch and touch the left elbow to the right knee. Keep up alternating sides in a bicycling-type motion. Repeat until you have touched each knee twenty times.

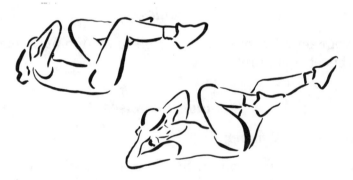

Stomach Crunch Number 3

While on your back, lift your head toward the ceiling with hands clasped behind the neck. With your legs crossed at the ankles, lift them in a bent position and let your elbows reach toward your knees. Twist the torso from side to side as your elbows reach for the opposite knee. Your legs should remain extended. Reach to each side twenty times.

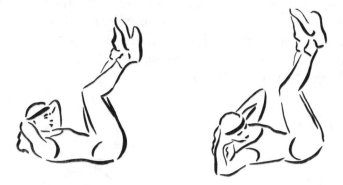

Torso Raises

Lie flat on your back with knees bent and arms straight by your side. With feet planted on the floor, about twelve inches apart, lift your torso as straight as possible. Repeat twenty times. Rest ten seconds and repeat twenty more times.

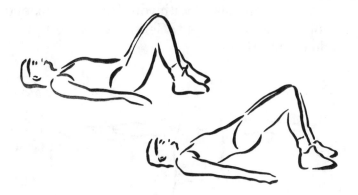

Cool Down Phase

Cooling down from exercise should not be skipped or rushed. It serves at least two important purposes. It gives your heart time to slow down gradually and gives you a chance to stretch out those muscles.

Sitting Stretch

Sit on the floor with legs extended and straight. Walk your hands down your legs as your back stretches and rounds over your legs. Reach for your toes. Pull forward keeping your legs straight. Do not bounce, just pull forward as far as possible and hold for a count of five. Repeat four more times.

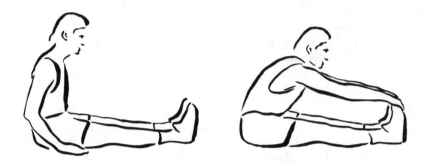

Back Release

Bend knees slightly and stand with your feet apart. Extend your arms straight out at shoulder height. Gently twist the upper body from side-to-side twenty times.

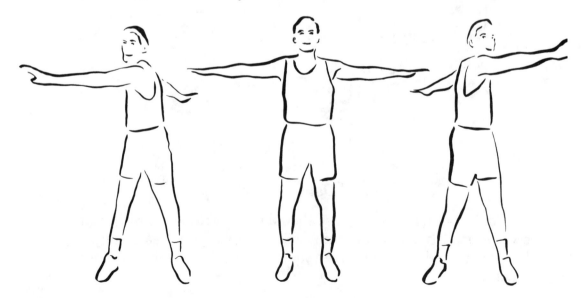

Neck Stretch

Stand tall with good posture and legs apart. Slowly rotate your head to the right, stopping when your ear is over your shoulder. Then, rotate to the left. Stretch your neck as far as you can four times on each side. Now slowly roll your head in circles toward the right four times and then toward the left four times.

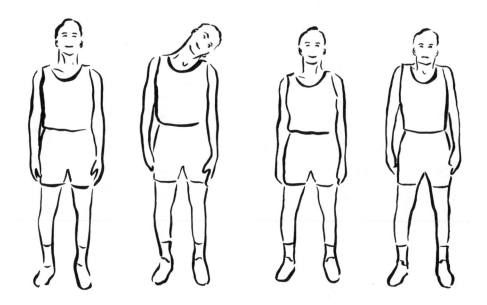

Shoulder Shrug

Continue standing with straight posture. Now raise your shoulders as high as possible and hold for three seconds as you breathe deeply. Roll your shoulders back down and breathe out. Repeat for a total of eight times.

Expect to steadily improve on your circuit-training program. Even though the exercise program is intense, you are doing aerobics and muscle toning simultaneously. You are making the most of your time. Push on to the next chapter, and let's discuss some of the most commonly asked questions in weight loss.

Weight Loss Q & A: Know the Real Facts

The following questions have been asked by actual patients over the last several years. I hope that the candor with which they are presented will help you with answers for your own dieting and weight-loss questions. Misinformation abounds in the world of nutrition since it is such big business. So keep these tidbits in mind when someone tries to take your time, money, and energy in return for some mythical cure for obesity.

The older I get, the less I seem able to lose weight. What's the problem?

After the age of twenty-five the resting metabolic rate (RMR) for humans decreases by 2 percent per decade on average. This makes it tougher to lose weight at sixty-five than at twenty-five or thirty-five. The sooner in life you get a handle on weight control, the better. But weight loss at any age is possible—just be patient with yourself and realize that a pound a week is progress.

The other reason for weight gain as we age is that our lean body mass (LBM) decreases as we get older. In fact, this is probably why our RMR decreases. So we need to try to continue or begin a fitness program that includes muscle-building as well as aerobics. This can be accomplished through the circuit-training course we presented in chapter 7.

I'm so hungry all the time. How can I stay on a diet when my hunger pangs are so intense?

If you are experiencing a lot of hunger, make an appointment with your physician to see if there is an underlying medical problem. Diabetes or hypoglycemia can often cause you to be hungrier than usual. Beyond that, avoid diets that severely restrict calories and opt for slower but steadier and more comfortable weight loss, such as the exchange diet in this book at the fourteen-hundred calorie level. This would be ideal for someone with hypoglycemia too.

A source of complete protein and adequate amounts of carbohydrates are essential for conquering hunger during fat reduction (for example, cottage cheese and fruit or a sandwich with lean meat). Also, increasing your fiber intake, drinking eight glasses of liquids a day, drinking hot liquids, and avoiding sugar will also help fill you up and stave off hunger.

Your physician can tell you whether or not you are a candidate for a appetite suppressant. Prescription medications, such as Fastin, can help you get started. They should not be taken for more than fourteen days in a row, however. I do not think the over-the-counter varieties are helpful. After your body becomes accustomed to less food, you will probably be less hungry.

Last, don't fall for fad diets! You are particularly vulnerable if you have had trouble losing weight in the past. They can only set you up for failure and convince you that you just can't lose weight.

What is cellulite? Will it go away as I lose weight?

Cellulite is nothing more than fat tissue that has popped out of the sheath that surrounds and separates it from the rest of the body. It is an inheritable trait. Though it often increases with age, you can see it in overfat younger people (even children). You can decrease cellulite by reducing your percent body fat through weight loss and aerobic exercise, which burns fat as a fuel source. Improving the tone of the underlying muscles will also smooth the appearance of cellulite.

PMS gets me each month. I will do great on controlled eating for two weeks and then do terrible for two weeks. How can I control my premenstrual hunger and urge for sweets?

Premenstrual syndrome (PMS) is alive and well and affects up to 90 percent of menstruating-age women. Increased hunger, bulimia, binges, and cravings for chocolate and sweets are a particular problem for some women who are severely affected each menstruating cycle. Also, feelings of hypoglycemia are common as part of PMS, and this can cause you to feel more fatigued and hungry than you normally would.

You must first determine if you have PMS, and you can only do this by journaling your symptoms on a special PMS chart as found in my book *PMS: What It Is and What You Can Do About It*, by Sneed and McIlhaney (Grand Rapids, Mich.: Baker Book House, 1988). An OB/GYN will tell you the same thing. It sometimes will take two or three menstrual-cycles to accurately diagnose PMS, and then another few cycles to weed through different treatment modalities to determine what is going to work for you.

If PMS is a significant problem, it is quite possible that you will lose weight for two weeks and then when you become premenstrual for the last two weeks of the cycle you will gain that weight back. I have had many patients between twenty-five and forty years of age that fall into this category.

PMS treatment revolves around aerobic exercise, weight loss, stress reduction, dietary changes (less salt, sugar, and caffeine), and appropriate medication. A few vitamin supplements may help, including vitamin B6.

Don't sit on this one. And don't settle for a physician intimating that it is all in your weak-willed mind. PMS is a real, physiological disorder and can make dieting very difficult until it is under control.

Are fresh-squeezed juices better for you than fresh fruits and vegetables? I've heard they can cure many ills, including headaches, arthritis, heart disease, hemorrhoids, and other health problems. They are also supposed to help you lose weight.

Many magazines and television ads would have you believe that you can get a lot more nutritive value from fruits and vegetables that have been put through an at-home juicer. They say that juices are better for you because they are more easily digested. In fact, liquids just leave the stomach faster than do solids, but solids will help you feel full and help stave off hunger.

Ounce for ounce, you will not get more nutrients with home-prepared juices, but you will substantially decrease the amount of fiber in your diet. I recommend whole fruits and vegetables as the mainstay and juices on occasion. In any case, there is certainly no need to purchase a costly juicer.

> *The health food store always seems to have dietary supplements and an endless stream of other get-slim-quick notions and potions, such as certain amino acid preparations, enzymes, and microbes like spirulina. Do any of these work?*

Health food shoppers are led to believe that weight loss may be bought instead of managed by a complete lifestyle program. Perhaps there will be a "magic pill" in the future that can help everyone be at the percentage body fat they desire. However, to date, there is no known material that can be added to a diet to cause body-fat reduction. Water loss can be achieved with any number of diuretics. And amphetamines can temporarily cause a reduction in appetite. But neither of these medications have been shown to aid in permanent weight loss.

> *Do vinegar and grapefruit have any place in weight reduction? I don't want to sound silly, but I have heard that they "melt" fat away.*

No food or pill can burn fat up. The old "grapefruit diet" was pushed many years ago, but it is clear that the acids that give vinegar and grapefruit their sour taste do not have the ability to burn up fat.

> *I have heard that protein is not fattening—in any quantity.*

Many foods high in protein are also high in fat. In fact, unless you are eating egg white, it is almost impossible to get totally fat-free and carbohydrate-free protein. Since fat supplies more than twice the amount of calories as protein and carbohydrate, excess amounts of protein should be avoided if for no other reason than keeping the fat intake down.

Should I give up red meats if I want to get weight off and keep it off for good?

Not at all. Red meat is so similar to our own nutritional needs for building muscle that it can supply many needed nutrients. Specifically, beef is high in iron, zinc, magnesium, and manganese. As we Americans have decreased our intake of beef, our intake in these important minerals has also decreased. Any of the "round" cuts such as round roast, eye of the round, round steak, or ground round (look for Healthy Choice™ ground round) are excellent sources of relatively lowfat protein, packed with other nutrients.

Should I be shopping at our local health food store more often? Should I buy only natural foods to avoid additives that I have heard can keep you from losing weight?

Don't be myth-taken on this one. You do not need special foods to stay healthy. You can get all the nutrients you need from foods at your regular grocery store. Some preservatives actually act as antioxidants, a general type of potential anticarcinogen that in other ways we seek through supplementation.

Foods may be labeled "natural," "organic," or may even say "health food." But the federal government has no legal definition for these terms. Thus, manufacturers can use these words to describe almost any product. They could be high in tropical oils and contain sixty percent fat and still be called "health food." Usually this term is used to up the selling price.

I began drinking juice by the quart when I was pregnant and never seemed to break the habit. Since it contains no fat, is it still okay to do this?

Apple juice is fifty-five calories for only one-half cup (or four ounces). Grape juice is even more calorie concentrated. Though juice has redeeming qualities and certainly tastes great, it is a source of both calories and sugar that I do not recommend for dieters. You are much better off to eat a whole fruit to fill an empty stomach than to quickly down some juice. Which do you think would make you feel more satisfied: one cup of ripe watermelon or one-half cup orange juice? Juice can still be worked into your diet plan, but is not as good a choice at this time as is whole fruit.

Juice is still a good choice for your children. If you are having trouble staying out of the juice bottle, though, try getting the small, individual serving cartons and let your children serve themselves.

Do you have any tips for someone on a very limited budget? I thought health foods were expensive.

"Health foods" from health food stores are indeed expensive. Fortunately, healthy foods from your grocery store are not. For protein sources, used dried beans (see meat alternatives), eggs, egg whites, tofu and buy round steak and other round cuts when they go on special. Go through the produce department buying what is in season and on special. Remember, there are no restrictions on vegetables and fruits in terms of what you can eat. Check your exchange lists to determine quantity and know with certainty that you may choose anything from the produce section and it can be worked into your diet.

For specialty items such as light bread, mayonnaise, and salad dressings, you may want to reserve these items for yourself— especially if you have children who are real calorie incinerators. Otherwise, eat what you cook for the rest of the family. Stay away from overt junk foods that can be very costly and are not good for anyone.

I have read in another diet book that you should not mix certain kinds of foods. For example, you should not eat protein with starch. Is there any truth to this? It makes going out to eat very difficult.

I hope you will continue to enjoy your grilled chicken breast with rice pilaf. There is absolutely not a hint of any information anywhere to substantiate these wild claims. When you hear research studies quoted, make sure you recognize the name of the organization or university conducting the research.

It is actually recommended that you eat a well-balanced meal with adequate amounts of carbohydrates, protein, and fat so that hunger pangs can be controlled for as long as possible.

If I control my salt and sodium intake, will I lose weight at a faster rate?

Sodium and salt restriction has only to do with water retention that will come and go according to what you have eaten for the day. One Chinese dinner could make you retain two pounds of water, and you could lose it the next day perspiring during a three-mile walk.

Salt restriction is only necessary (1) if you really eat too many salty things, (2) if you have high blood pressure, or (3) when PMS and premenstrual water retention is a real problem. Otherwise, restriction of salt will not help you lose fat, though it is an overall good health habit.

My biggest problems seem to center around spouse sabotage. Ice cream, chips, and everything is brought into the house by persons other than myself. Then I find that I can't resist them. What can I do?

It is the special spouse who does everything right for the would-be dieter. Weight can often be a source of emotional friction in the intimate relationship of marriage. This makes it difficult to talk about and "clear the air." Some spouses will feel convicted themselves when you begin to diet, knowing that it is high time for them to make the same choices. Or perhaps they are bitter because you have not been successful at weight loss in the past. Others feel threatened that they will now be forced to eat "diet food." I want to go on record here as saying there is no such thing as diet food. There is only healthy food or unhealthy food; and all adults need the same type of healthy food, no matter what they weigh.

The only thing you can do when living with others and trying to diet is to ask them for their help in a loving way. Do not be hateful, resentful, or unkind. Don't make accusations or blame them for things. Most people can't resist kindness, and sometimes it is even contagious. Other than this, I have no other suggestions.

You say that this is a diet that the whole family can enjoy. Does that mean that even children can follow this style of eating program?

Absolutely. Past the age of two, no one needs much fat in their diet. Keep children on whole milk (unless they are obese) until they are two. Meanwhile, buy everyone else skimmed milk or ½ percent milk. When the child turns two, you may then give everyone the same of everything. The exceptions are these: (1) Nutrasweet and other artificial sweeteners are not recommended for children and pregnant women; (2) those at a normal weight do not need light breads (forty-calorie variety); (3) extra calories for growing teens should be provided with extra complex carbohydrates after all other nutritional needs have been met.

Keep this in mind too—children are teachable. Over two years of age, intensive dietary counseling has been shown in research studies to decrease the fat intake of children and cause a reduction in relative weight in obese children aged six to sixteen. Believe it or not, my own kids are checking for fat in foods sometimes, raising an eyebrow if they have been given something that is not a healthy choice.

It seems like when I regain weight now it comes back in less flattering places, like my lower abdomen. Is there something to this, or is it just my imagination?

As we age, both men and women tend to collect more fat in the abdominal area. This is particularly true if your weight has gone down and then is regained. Fat seems to be added in this area the quickest, but is often lost from this area in the initial dieting stages as well.

I am having a hard time breaking away from some of my old favorites, like French fries and burgers, candy bars and so forth. Am I doomed to miss these things forever?

There are lower calorie and lower fat alternatives for almost all foods. You must be prepared to make a commitment that old items are eaten infrequently, but the lower fat alternatives may be eaten routinely. For example, try the hamburger and fries alternative listed on page 000. With these recipes you can actually have a full-sized burger and homemade steak fries for less than four hundred calories.

Or choose a granola bar instead of a candy bar. Learn to make low-calorie brownies (page 224). How about a lowfat serving of strawberry shortcake instead of a slice of uninspired bakery cake? These are the kinds of choices you must learn to make as a routine part of your management program.

Can I ever be as thin as I was in my late teens and early twenties?

Anyone can lose to a certain weight with enough calorie restriction. But at what price? As we get older, our lean body mass has a natural tendency to decrease while our percent body fat increases. Also, our basal metabolic rate (BMR) decreases slightly with each passing decade. All these small factors add up to the fact that it is often very difficult to maintain the exact weight of those earlier days. The important thing is to keep your weight at a comfortable and healthy weight for you now. Don't drive yourself crazy and succumb to irrational dieting fads in an attempt to regain youth. It will make you miserable.

After my weight is off, can I occasionally enjoy some of the old rich foods, like a piece of pie, cake, or candy?

That really depends on what you call occasionally. Does that mean only a few times per year, once a month, or weekly? It only takes one hundred extra calories per day to make your body gain ten pounds of fat in a year. If you go back to two desserts per week that your body does not burn up, that may be enough to cause the added weight gain.

Before you take that next bite of "a little something extra," consider the "Time/Activity Required to Burn Certain Foods" chart on page 176.

What is the best way to get rid of stretch marks?

There is really not much you can do about these. Stretch mark creams may make them temporarily less noticeable but cannot remove them. Known to doctors as *striae distensae*, stretch marks often occur as a result of weight gain or pregnancy (and even in weightlifters, particularly if they use steroids).

Stretch marks are a mild form of scarring that occurs when the

Time/Activity Required to Burn Certain Foods

Food	Minutes of Activity		
	Fast Walking	Biking	Jogging
½ cup ice cream	24	15	12
1 oz. cheese	22	13	11
1 slice cake with icing	100	63	50
2 oz. chocolate candy bar	60	38	30
1 doughnut	50	31	25
1 slice apple pie	90	64	45
1 slice pecan pie	150	94	75
12 oz. soft drink (not diet)	30	19	15
mayonnaise, 1 Tbsp.	20	12	10

connective tissue is stretched beyond its capacity. Heredity also seems to play a role in who gets stretch marks and who does not. For example, not all pregnant women get them.

One recent study has shown that the application of Retin-A (the trade name for tretinoin, a vitamin A derivative sold by prescription only) was helpful in all but one case. Some patients had complete clearing of the marks, but we still don't know if this is a permanent fix.

Retin-A may produce side effects such as red, swollen, and peeling skin and is also known to produce birth defects. *Retin-A should not be used by pregnant or nursing women.* The good news is that most stretch marks tend to fade in coloration with time. This may be the best course of action.

Do excess pounds on different areas of the body pose any different health threats?

Research indicates that the "spare tire" created by excess fat around the abdomen poses a particularly high hazard to health because it raises the risk of developing heart disease and diabetes. Where the body stores fat can be just as important to your health as how many pounds are stored.

To check your body shape, measure your waist while standing

relaxed, without pulling in your stomach. Then measure your hips around the buttocks, where they are the largest. Finally divide your waist measurement by the hip measurement to determine your waist-to-hip ratio. Ideally, the ratio should be less than one. In fact 0.80 or less is the target for women. They tend to have proportionately smaller waists and larger hips than men, who should aim for no more than 0.95. Beyond these cutoff points, the higher the number the greater the risk of health problems.

If I really want to lose weight, should I eliminate cakes, cookies, ice cream, and candy as a first line of offense?

Granted, because cake, cookies, and the like typically contribute lots of fat and calories to the diet and few other nutrients, it makes sense for the person on a weight-loss regimen to cut back on those foods. Nevertheless, the belief that to lose weight it is necessary to swear off sugar altogether is erroneous.

The first step in creating a successful weight-loss plan is identifying dietary changes that you can make comfortably. Some people go "cold turkey" and eliminate (at least for awhile) particular foods they find hard to stop eating once they have started. The bottom line, though, is that there is no one diet that will help everyone to shed pounds. You must find the system that is just right for you within certain guidelines. There is nothing inherently wrong with having some sugar in your diet if that's what it takes to set up a program you can live with.

I consider myself to be a good cook and am doing many of the lowfat things you have suggested in this book. I meticulously trim fat from all meat products. Am I still getting any cholesterol in my diet?

Cholesterol is found in the meat's lean as well as fatty tissue. It is in the cells of all animals (meat or fish), and the foods derived from them (butter, cheese, eggs, and milk). Needless to say, they are present in varying quantities. Still, you have earned your healthy-cooking chef's hat by eliminating fat where you see it. Fat contains loads of saturated fat that can turn into cholesterol in your body. Ultimately, it is best to choose lean, well-trimmed portions and then eat moderate amounts of animal products as listed in this book.

I have several mouths to feed in my family, and I usually like to buy the ground beef that says 75 percent lean. Doesn't that mean it is 25 percent fat, and thus it is on my diet?

No, in fact, this meat would be very fatty and the label is deceptive. It is 25 percent fat by weight. Remember that fat weighs less than lean meat (see page 13). A pan-fried patty of the meat (four ounces before cooking, three ounces after) would have about 260 calories and nineteen grams of fat. An equal serving size of ground round (I recommend that you buy Healthy Choice™ ground round) would only be in the 140-calorie range. In the end, you should give your family less meat, more complex carbohydrates, and less fat. You will not spend any more money in doing this. Think about how much cooks out of poor quality hamburger. Ground round is the only reasonable choice in choosing ground beef. (Don't let them grind up any extra fat in your ground round either.)

Are the cheeses made with part-skimmed milk okay to use on an everyday basis?

Not necessarily. Ricotta and mozzarella are the most common part-skim cheeses. You do save a few calories and grams of fat by using these versions, but look at the chart below to see if they fit into your diet plan. As with other higher fat foods, they should be used sparingly.

	Calories	Fat (g)	% Calories From Fat
Mozzarella, whole-milk, 1 oz.	80	6	68
Mozzarella, part-skim, 1 oz.	72	4.5	56
Ricotta, whole-milk, ½ cup	216	16	67
Ricotta, part-skim, ½ cup	171	10	53

Ever since I had kids, I have this disgusting fat over my lower abdomen. I'm desperate. What if I made a commitment to do five thousand sit-ups a month—would that take care of my problem?

There is no such thing as spot reducing. You can't do sit-ups and expect to lose the fat over the abdomen just as you can't do leg-lifts and expect to lose fat off the thighs. Calorie restriction and calorie burning exercise helps to lose fat over the entire body.

However, having strong abdominal muscles is always a plus. They will help you with every other activity you do and will tone the muscle area underneath the fat for a smooth appearance once the fat is gone.

Is margarine always better for you than butter?

Not necessarily, since margarine contains hydrogenated fats. The normally liquid unsaturated vegetable oils that make up margarine are altered by the process of hydrogenation: the addition of hydrogen atoms solidifies the fatty acids, makes them more saturated, and also turns some of them into "trans fats." A recent study found that trans fats can cause blood levels of cholesterol to rise, though not as much as saturated fats (the kind found in butter). It's true that margarine doesn't contain any cholesterol, which is an advantage; but it does have the same amount of fat and calories as butter. So, choose whichever you prefer and eat as little as possible of these high-fat foods.

I eat popcorn all the time now. At least I gave up chips. Did I make a good decision in doing this? I live alone and usually just use a pop-in-the-bag product. Are these alright to use?

That depends upon which product you are using and how much of it you eat. I am going to assume that very few people will pop a bag of corn and then save half for tomorrow. Some bagged popcorn contains up to four hundred calories per bag and still claims to contain no butter. The best choice is something like Smartfood™ Light Butter popcorn at thirty-five calories per cup and only 140 calories for the whole bag. Though it still contains six grams of fat, it takes care of the calorie and quantity problem. Otherwise, see page 226 for a lowfat and easy way to make your own light popcorn at home.

I want to quit smoking, but I am afraid I will gain even more weight. What can I do? Is there really a connection between the two?

"Reach for a Lucky Instead of a Sweet" was an actual 1920s advertising slogan that played on a "flapper's" desire to be ultra slim. Dr. Elliot Winebeurg, a smoking cessation expert, contends that most women smokers still make a conscious effort to smoke so that they can maintain their weight. This is phenomenal, since cigarette smoking is responsible for 30 percent of all cancers, with lung cancer being the number-one killer of women.

There are three probable reasons smokers gain weight. First, they often change their eating patterns, including an increase in the amount of food consumed. Second, they often will crave comfort foods to help them through tobacco withdrawal. Third, the metabolism may decrease slightly with the disappearance of nicotine. All of these things may be counteracted by a tobacco-abstinence program that can help you deal with these issues. Smoking is your number-one health risk. Find the motivation to quit this addiction through local programs, the American Cancer Society, or your local physician.

Can I just eat one meal a day and forget everything else in order to lose weight?

People who skip breakfast and lunch, eating only one meal a day, have the lowest metabolic rates compared to people who eat more frequently. In addition, these meal skippers overcompensate for the calories skipped and end up eating more than they would have if they had eaten the previous meals. Next are those who eat only two meals per day. People who eat three meals a day have the highest metabolic rates. Your metabolic rate rises after each meal and burns off much of what you have eaten. Eating more than three meals a day does not have any additional beneficial effects, however. A person who eats more than three meals per day does not experience much of a rise in metabolic rate and may consume excess calories unless snacks are quite small and low in calories.

Why does my stomach growl? It is a really embarrassing problem for me when I am on a diet.

The gurgling noises occur only when air or other gases are present in your digestive tract. Muscles in the walls of the digestive tract move the mixture of partially digested food and digestive juices along in a process called peristalsis. You are more likely to hear this noise when you're hungry because you tend to salivate more then and swallow more air. Try drinking water to quell some of this noise.

I can always count on myself to lose twenty pounds and then I seem to just stall out or "plateau." What does that really mean and what causes it?

The "plateau" in dieting is nothing more than your body being in a state of flux. After you have lost twenty pounds, it takes a further restriction of calories for you to lose more weight. If a man began this diet weighing 200 pounds and then lost to 180, he has less weight and work to do each day by virtue of the fact that he is carrying around twenty fewer pounds with every step. When in an actual state of weight loss, the metabolic rate is also temporarily and slightly depressed.

Beyond preparing yourself with this knowledge, you can also do two things. First, step up your exercise by one hour per week. Also, consider cutting your caloric intake by one hundred calories per day and seriously examine whether you are returning to old ways. This is a dangerous point for any dieter. It is often a decision-making point where we determine whether these changes are temporal or permanent.

150 Action Tips for Permanent Weight Loss

Here we are nearing the end of another weight-loss book. But this time you sense that you are going to follow through. You realize this is a sensible program that has life-changing potential. It is not a fly-by-night fad diet book you will sell for fifty cents in your next garage sale. It is a different sort of program, and by now maybe you are different too.

The following action steps are a compilation of many things we have discussed in greater detail in this book, and other helpful suggestions. They are not in any particular order to illustrate the necessity of a "whole body" approach to weight loss. Dwell on these steps. Live by them. And then, add some new steps of your own.

1. Be joyful for who you are. God loves you. You need to love yourself as well. Be positive about your diet and your body.

2. Enlist a friend as a dieting confidant. Have them check your food diaries (like the one on page 44) and perhaps even your weight once every two weeks.

3. Take a packet of low-cal salad dressing, like Skinny Haven, and a shaker of butter substitute, like Molly McButter, in your purse or satchel when you know that you will eat a salad and baked potato at a restaurant. It will save you up to six hundred calories of pure fat.

4. Get a dog so you will feel compelled to take it on walks.

5. Make a conscious effort not to let significant others make you believe that you will fail on this diet because there have been other diet failures in the past. Many of the other diets set you up for failure.

6. Choose to live.

7. Enjoy grilled cheese sandwiches with your kids using lite bread and lite cheese (see page 230). They will love it, and so will you (up to four hundred calories saved).

8. Go to the movies with no money other than the admission fee to help you get rid of the movie popcorn urge. Put a canned diet drink from home in your pocket in case you are tempted to take money for a drink and in the end, opt for another selection. You can probably take in your own lowfat popcorn too. Most movies will let you bring something in if you tell them you are on a special diet.

9. When going out to lunch or dinner, plan what you will eat before you arrive. Mention it to someone in casual conversation.

10. Cut back on your living expenses enough so that you can work less and take time for at least four hours per week of aerobic exercise.

11. Buy a real bicycle. They are great fun and are not just for kids. I find them less boring than stationary varieties. Wear a helmet.

12. Establish rewards for yourself for every ten-pound weight loss. Stick by these guidelines. Don't buy anything until the weight is lost—not even if it goes on sale.

13. Take some gourmet cooking classes that focus on lowfat foods and recipes.

14. Find some new friends who enjoy good health and healthy activities.

15. Find another health-conscious friend who would like to be a walking buddy. It will give you a sense of security and commitment.

16. Order spaghetti with marinara sauce in Italian restaurants instead of Fettucini Alfredo or Eggplant Parmesan.

17. When eating in a Mexican food restaurant, lay five tortilla chips in front of you and eat them slowly. Don't go back for more. Make a point of setting the basket on the other side of the table or have the waiter remove it altogether.

18. If you are walking twelve miles per week or more, you should probably replace your walking shoes every six to eight months.

19. Forgive someone today. Grudges don't do anyone any good.

20. Try a new lowfat recipe once a week from your local newspaper, magazines, and cookbooks until you have a repertoire of "good eats" for every occasion.

21. Next time you take a plane trip, order the lowfat or low-calorie special dinner. These usually contain better food choices anyway.

22. Consider a new hairstyle as you lose your weight.

23. Join an audio book club in your area. Tapes are great companions for your walking/jogging time.

24. Realize there is a limit to things that can be demanded of you. You should have at least an hour per day all to yourself for prayer, exercise, and peace of mind. Work toward this goal.

25. Love your spouse. If you feel your relationship needs a tune-up, go to a marriage conference. They are great for helping to restore "the old zing." Remember, your first familial commitment should be to your spouse—not your children. Two organizations you can call are any Minirth-Meier clinic in your area or Here's Life America (look in the phone book).

26. If you are living with a member of the opposite sex out of wedlock, ask yourself if this type of noncommittal attitude is what you really want out of life. Doesn't commitment through thick and thin sound better than maybe? Don't let this mixed-up world tell you what is right. Listen to your heart.

27. Do a kind deed for someone once a week. There are people out there in droves who need you! Remember, according to the family practice doctors, a necessary part of the formula for the happy adult is to help others.

28. Order just the right amount of pizza so that there will neither be too much nor will there be leftovers. Order peppers, onion, mushrooms, or Canadian bacon as alternatives to sausage and pepperoni.

29. Buy yourself some good cookware that is fun to use. Make sure a vegetable steamer comes with the set.

30. Take dancing lessons. Go as a couple or try a singles class. Community colleges are fun and inexpensive ways to start. I would put a good polka or Texas two-step up against any aerobics class.

31. Keep your house relatively orderly, but don't expect perfection from yourself or anyone else. There is no such thing as perfection in this world.

32. Be the first to order at a restaurant. Don't wait for your friends to choose incorrectly and influence your decision making.

33. Never buy holiday candies in advance. Buy them a few hours before you need them and do not overbuy. Send leftovers home with someone else.

34. Don't ever wear exercise clothing that makes you sweat unduly. Choose exercise clothes that are cool and comfortable and let air circulate around your skin.

35. If you do not know how, learn to swim; and then use this as part of your exercise program.

36. As Tina Turner said at age fifty-two, "What has age got to do with it?" It is never too early or too late to be healthy.

37. Do not return to restaurants in which you consistently make poor choices.

38. Don't be surprised, humiliated, or demoralized when you have dieting setbacks. I think of food addiction recovery as many alcoholics think of sobriety. A part of me will always know how to bury problems underneath food, but I can count how many years it has been since I have actually behaved in this way.

39. Use nonstick cooking sprays and nonstick cookware to save hundreds of calories from most cooked recipes.

40. If you are an afternoon grazer while you are cooking for the rest of the family, cook your evening meal in the morning as you clean up the breakfast dishes. Refrigerate until ready to heat for supper.

41. Do not ever buy anything at the grocery store that is a nutritionally poor choice simply because it is "a good deal."

42. Next time you buy a new car, swear off letting anyone (yourself included) bring food into the car. If you are not going to buy a new car, treat yourself to a great car wash and then do the same.

43. Do not buy or cook treats for the rest of the family that you know you cannot resist yourself. At some point there has to be an end of it. If these foods are not good for you, they are not good for the rest of the family either.

44. If you are doing fine with your diet at work except for the candy machine in the afternoon, do not take any money to work. Take credit cards for an emergency and one quarter for a phone call. Leave

the rest of your money at home. You will be tempted to borrow once; I doubt if you will do it twice, however.

45. Avoid eating at your desk at work at any time. Working with food in your hand can get to be an associated habit, which is hard to break—especially if your job becomes stressful.

46. Do a minimum of fifteen minutes of calisthenics every day just to keep your body feeling good.

47. Make it a practice to never buy food, cookies, or candies from cute kids who show up on your doorstep. One box of cookies in a lonely apartment or house can destroy the emotional and physical progress you have made over the last month.

48. Are you willing to walk as much as seven miles to burn off a piece of pecan pie you can eat in only three minutes? Instead, try a large serving of fresh strawberries and lite Cool Whip for one hundred guilt-free calories.

49. Pick up a good book (like this one!) every few months and be prepared to tell someone about what you are reading.

50. If you are a TV addict, work on giving it up. Fill your life with other things. Profuse and mindless television watching is a death-blow for your new eating and lifestyle. Schedule specific programs you would like to watch. Don't just "see what's on."

51. If you are watching television during mealtimes, this must go—even if you live alone. The association between food and TV is too powerful to ignore.

52. A maintenance program is simply that. It means you maintain the good habits you have already begun.

53. You will almost always gain back a few pounds once you complete a diet. Lose a few more pounds than really needed to prepare for this event.

54. Avoid friends who were former "eating buddies" for the first month of your new diet.

55. Every twelve-ounce serving of diet soda contains the equivalent of six packages of Equal. I recommend no more than two twelve-ounce diet sodas per day.

56. If you get that urge for a cheeseburger and fries, make use of the suggested recipes on page 225 and save yourself about three hundred to four hundred calories of almost pure fat.

57. Learn to control rebellion against restrictions. No one really has it "their own way" all the time.

58. Prepare a snack box for your children and your husband, which contains fruits, dried fruits, snack packages, light cupcakes, and so forth. They can choose snacks out of the box so that the food never has to touch your hands. The more you are exposed to food, the more you will be tempted to nibble.

59. Never overstock or overbuy perishable food items. When they start to go bad, we tend to increase our eating to keep pace.

60. Avoid taking items to potluck dinners and other social gatherings that you cannot eat. You will be tempted to snack during the preparation process and at the event itself. There are alternatives for almost any recipe. Take these instead.

61. Ask someone for a food processor for Christmas. It is an essential item. (Get a good one.)

62. Over the age of two, everyone in the house may eat the lowfat way. Children aged three and older may use skimmed milk, lowfat cheeses, and all other foods and recipes recommended for you. One exception is that they should not consume Nutrasweet™.

63. Cook meals for the entire family based around your new eating program. Do not prepare separate meals for everyone else. Use rec-

ipes in the back of the *Love Hunger* book—such as meat loaf, mashed potatoes, enchiladas, and chicken jambalaya—which won't make anyone feel like they are on a diet.

64. Tell a few people you are on a weight-reduction program, but don't tell everyone.

65. Make a commitment to exercise at least four hours per week for the rest of your life. Experts continue to agree that this is one of the greatest factors in keeping weight off. It should be a lifelong ritual you learn to enjoy.

66. Look for exercise activities you enjoy, like tennis, racquetball, dancing, and mountain biking. If you don't enjoy exercise, you won't keep it up.

67. At holiday times, never give cookies and candies as gifts. This is often a convenient excuse to have these items in your house. And you are modeling a tradition for your children they may feel obligated to continue.

68. Holiday gift alternatives for friends and neighbors include potpourri, homemade ornaments and knickknacks, homemade barbecue sauce, homemade jams and jellies, homemade breads (yeast varieties). All are preferable to high-fat cookies, cakes, and candies.

69. Purchase a small and insulated lunch container that can accommodate diet sodas or other drinks, fruits, and sandwiches, or other main course material to take to work with you. Leave the rest of your money at home.

70. Drink at least eight to ten glasses of liquid, tea, or diet sodas per day. At least half of this should be water.

71. An easy way to encourage yourself to drink more water at work is to keep an insulated cup of ice water on your desk and drink one in the morning and one in the afternoon.

72. Remember grocery store rules, like never go to the store when you are hungry or look for something you should not have. Go for a walk first, have a light snack, and wait for your mood to be more positive.

73. Don't ever think of walking time as time that is wasted. During this thirty to sixty minutes per day you may learn a foreign language, listen to motivational tapes (like *Love Hunger* on tape), listen to a novel, sermons, or any number of other audio tapes available at local libraries and bookstores.

74. Always keep extra batteries for your walkman on hand. Indulge in a good walkman cassette player.

75. When you sit down to a meal, concentrate on eating slowly, drinking a lot of water, and engaging in conversation if you are dining with someone else. Lay your fork down whenever possible. Linger over a long, cool glass of iced tea or water with a twist of lemon or lime.

76. Though in the initial stages of research, *limene*, one of the essential elements of limes, has been found to be an anticarcinogen (cancer-preventing chemical) in laboratory tests. Iced water with a twist of fresh lime is a very fresh-tasting, non-caloric beverage.

77. The vast majority of lifestyle changes you make to lose weight also help to prevent cancer, high blood pressure, heart disease, and diabetes.

78. Even though complex carbohydrates are good for us all (if there is not much added fat), the larger quantities should only be in your diet if you are working out consistently and engaged in endurance sports.

79. Arrange your closet from the largest sizes down to the smallest sizes, not seasonally. Wear the things you can now, and as you lose weight, have them altered or discard them altogether. As the old out-

fits leave your wardrobe, see what new size is next in line to be worn.

80. Don't buy clothes that don't fit in anticipation of losing the weight. Instead, buy an item that fits and looks flattering to you as a reward for reaching a certain goal. You should have perks and prizes for yourself along the way as various weight goals are reached.

81. Rewards every ten pounds might include clothes, perfume, make-overs, a personal item, or something for your home that you have wanted for some time. At the end of your weight loss, consider giving yourself a big trip or the equivalent.

82. If you are not part of a local weight-loss or therapy group, consider finding a friend and confidant who has the same goals in mind as you do. Together you can weigh, go through the book, share recipes, walk, and promote other positive new changes. You might even plan a vacation together (with spouses if applicable) to celebrate reaching your goal weight.

83. Make sure to get rid of fitted clothes (like blue jeans) that are too large and too difficult to alter.

84. At the most, weigh once a week. Every two weeks is better. If you weigh every day, you will become discouraged watching the standard pair of bathrom scales inch down. Even if you lose one-quarter of a pound (which is undetectable on many scales), you have lost a stick of butter.

85. If you see yourself beginning to lose control, go back to using a food journal.

86. Remove or store all visible food in your house. Don't leave anything sitting out (including a fruit bowl) that could cause you to grab something as you walk by that you would not otherwise have taken.

87. Never cut out coupons for foods that are poor food choices. If the food is something you and your family do not need, it is not a bargain at any price.

88. Walk at the nearest mall on rainy days instead of missing your exercise altogether.

89. Lowfat gravies may be made and used at any time. Use skimmed milk and flour (mixed cold) for a creamed gravy and defatted pan drippings or bouillon (cold) mixed with flour for brown gravy. Season; thicken by boiling and serve as often as you like.

90. When you have a shorter time than usual for your exercise time, you can use one-pound ankle weights and carry small hand weights to get a more intensive workout in a shorter length of time.

91. Also on busy days, keep in mind that household duties can be aerobic, including mopping, mowing the lawn, vacuuming, and walking quickly to the corner market or dry cleaners.

92. Think of all the money you are spending on junk food. Every time you save a few dollars by avoiding the convenience store or candy machine, save it in an envelope that will serve as money to be spent on rewards for yourself at every ten-pound loss.

93. If you have small children at home, do not feel that exercise is not an option for you. Consider a Gerry carrier or a stroller that is meant for fast walking. A woman in my neighborhood used to faithfully take her triplets in a stroller built for three for one hour each day. It was uphill too.

94. If you do not consistently have two or three servings per day of a skimmed milk product, you should take a calcium supplement.

95. Get a medical checkup before beginning a diet. Go back and request blood work for every thirty-pound loss.

96. Menstruating-age women are particularly susceptible to anemia, especially if they are eating less red meat (which is high in iron). If you are feeling tired, talk to your doctor and have blood work done to determine whether you are anemic.

97. If you do not have an open mind about new foods and recipes, none of this will ever stick. Remember, the old ways are not an option anymore.

98. Never volunteer to consistently work around food (such as being refreshment coordinator for a women's group). The temptation will be too great, and you can serve in other capacities.

99. Get passionate about something in your life. Take up a new hobby, civic project, or new job.

100. When you begin to feel overstressed, seek help from whomever you can to ease your workload. Also eliminate things from your "to do" list as soon as possible, and get your life back in order quickly. Overstressed people do not have the time or inclination to take care of themselves properly. Nor, can they be successful dieters.

101. When you make casseroles, soups, stews, chili, or other freezable meals (even hamburger patties), make enough for an extra meal or two. By freezing the extras, you will be exposed to food less often. Working with food causes us all to nibble. Get into a habit of not eating while you cook, but also cook less often.

102. Package smaller leftovers with a purpose in mind, such as lunch tomorrow. Then you will be less likely to munch on that extra half cup of rice as you clean the kitchen.

103. Clean up the dishes immediately after eating, as opposed to letting leftovers sit out for an hour or two. In two hours you might be hungry enough to eat the leftovers instead of packaging them. It will also cut down on spoilage.

104. Happy people make successful dieters. If you are unhappy much of the time, see your doctor. Find out if you might have clinical depression, situational depression, PMS, or some other medical reason for dissatisfaction.

105. Never start a diet when you are under unbearable stress. Take a

week off to get a good start, plan meals, enjoy low-cal cooking, and walk, walk, walk.

106. Don't ignore skimmed-milk products in your daily diet. You don't absorb calcium or phosophorous as well from a supplement as you do from the real thing. It is also very filling, low in calories and fat, high in protein, and can be used in many wonderful recipes.

107. Would you rather have one peanut butter and jelly sandwich on standard bread for 350 calories or two tuna sandwiches made with forty-calorie bread and lite mayonnaise for three hundred calories?

108. Be realistic about your rate of weight loss. Having unrealistic expectations can ruin your momentum. Expect no more than a three-pound-per-week loss when you are far from your goal and perhaps a one-pound-per-week loss when you are closer to your goal.

109. Women who watch TV more than four hours per day are twice as likely to be obese compared to those who watch less than two hours per day. TV watching increases snacking and decreases time spent in exercise. Earlier studies have shown this same relationship to be true for children.

110. To burn up four Hershey's kisses, it takes fifteen to twenty minutes of walking, twelve minutes of bike riding, or ten minutes of swimming or jogging.

111. Caffeine and alcohol can sometimes act as appetite stimulants. Try to determine if they make you hungrier. If they do, avoid them.

112. *Consumer Reports* (May 1992) lists the Saucony Jazz 3000 as the best quality and best buy in a jogging/running shoe. They cost about half as much as some of their counterparts.

113. If you have maturity-onset diabetes, elevated cholesterol, or high serum triglycerides, chances are great that they will normalize or at least normalize to some degree as you lose weight. We have

patients in our practice who have been able to do away with medications for diabetes, high blood pressure, depression, and high cholesterol by losing weight and consistently exercising. Always check with your doctor. Don't make these pharmaceutical changes on your own.

114. There is such a keen relationship between obesity and disease that if the entire population of the United States were at optimal body weight, it has been estimated that the coronary heart disease incidence could be reduced by 25 percent and congestive heart failure and stroke by thirty-five percent. A fifteen percent decline in mortality would be seen overall.

115. The risk of developing diabetes among people forty-five to seventy-four years of age more than doubles with every twenty-percent excess in body weight. If obesity were not present in the United States, type II diabetes (maturity-onset) could be reduced by 50 percent.

116. Weight loss is the first line of treatment of obese patients with type II diabetes, elevated serum cholesterol or triglyceride levels, and those patients with high blood pressure.

117. Experts agree that exercise is the critical factor in not regaining weight that has been lost.

118. When weight is lost and then regained, it is more difficult to lose the same weight again. More calories must be restricted the second time around in order to lose the same amount of weight. Roller-coaster dieting may work for a few years during youth, but sooner or later, you'll be at the top and won't be able to get down.

119. Anticipate snacks that you will need throughout the day and take them in your car or keep them in your office. A nice juicy apple makes a great snack that will help you feel light and full of energy. Convenience stores offer very little in the way of nutritious snack options.

120. If a food leaves a grease spot on a napkin, it is generally high in fat. Foods that fit this description include crackers, cookies, baked goods, muffins, cheeses, chips, and fried foods.

121. Think of food as fuel for your body. When your tanks are full, there's no need to top them off.

122. New evidence from Johns Hopkins University School of Medicine show that broccoli contains a compound known as *sulforaphane*. This chemical may trigger increased production of special enzymes in the body's cells that ward off cancer-causing agents. Cooked, chopped broccoli is only twenty-three calories per half cup serving. This vegetable packs more nutrition and benefits per calorie than almost any other food. Use it frequently.

123. Other vegetables of the cruciferous family (broccoli family) that may contain cancer-fighting agents are Brussels sprouts, cabbage, mustard greens, kale, kohlrabi, and cauliflower. They are all low in calories.

124. Making Jello pudding (any cook-and-serve flavor) with skimmed milk yields a product that is only 130 calories per one-half cup serving. It is a great family pleaser and is good for your children too. For diabetes, try the sugar-free varieties made with skimmed milk for a product that is only ninety calories per serving and no fat.

125. Remember to pack some great-tasting and nutritious snacks for the family when going on a trip. Don't count on finding a good choice at convenience stores.

126. One of the biggest keys to successful weight maintenance for life is to achieve a muscular body composition. You cannot maintain or gain muscle without exercise.

127. The only diet foods you should ever consider are those that can someday be modified for a permanent eating plan by adding larger portions and a few more food choices.

128. When seeking an expert in your own geographical area to help you with nutrition information, choose a registered dietitian (R.D.).

129. Do you take at least twenty minutes to finish your food? Remember that this amount of time is required in order for the food you eat to reach the hunger center in your brain and turn off the hunger switch. If you eat quickly (in ten minutes, for example), you might eat a large meal and still be hungry. At these times you may be tempted to add something else to your meal because you think you have not had enough food. Instead, give it a few more minutes and your hunger will disappear.

130. My most successful patients at the clinic were ones who kept a daily food diary and were accountable to themselves for the food they ate. Food diaries are a way that we come to terms with just how much we are eating.

131. The best food diary is one you can carry in a pocket and take with you everywhere. Wear clothes that contain pockets, and let it be a constant reminder that if you pick up a little something here and there, you have to "fess up" in the diary. See page 44 if you want a more structured food diary.

132. You can usually see your clothes fit better on a daily basis. Use this as a daily gauge and weigh yourself weekly.

133. Sugary foods cause you to become hungry shortly after eating them. However, complex carbohydrates and proteins help you to stave off hunger four times longer than sugar. So try to include a protein source in every snack as well as meals. Cottage cheese and fruit is a nice way to combine these two nutrients.

134. How can you identify a three-ounce portion when eating out? It is the size of a lady's hand, the amount commonly on a sandwich, the amount on a "quarter pounder," half a chicken breast, or what we commonly call the meat-portion size on the "light plate" at a cafeteria.

135. If you leave off the cheese and mayonnaise from a hamburger, you have just cut almost two hundred calories of pure fat.

136. The grilled chicken sandwich at many fast food restaurants is the best fast food choice if you have them cut the mayonnaise and cheese. The Chicken Fajita Pita at Jack-in-the-Box is also very low in fat.

137. Peanut butter is like spreading on regular butter with a little added protein. It is almost pure fat. Is this really what you want in your body?

138. A Dannon light yogurt that is nonfat and sweetened with Nutrasweet™ is a good choice at snacktime or for dessert.

139. Don't forget popsicles and frozen fruit bars for a summertime treat. There are many natural versions that are made from real fruits and contain no artificial additives. Calorie values for these range from seventeen to one hundred. Almost all of these are no fat or low-fat.

140. You must walk up thirty flights of stairs to burn up one small handful of nuts (one oz.) having 180 calories of almost pure fat. All nuts are very high in fat. Macadamia nuts are 95 percent fat. None are a good choice for munching. Use them sparingly in cooking.

141. Stretching before and after exercise sessions helps you avoid injury. Don't neglect this important part of your workout.

142. Eliminate dabs and dollops of butter on top of casseroles. You will probably find that you do not miss them.

143. Make soups and stews frequently. If you can make them ahead of time, you can refrigerate and lift off any fat that is present after it has hardened.

144. Soups are an excellent way to incorporate more vegetables into the diet for non-vegetable lovers. They are usually low in calories and fat, and hot liquids serve as appetite quenchers.

145. Season vegetables with herbs, spices, broths, and bouillon cubes instead of animal fat or butter. There is no place for cooking with bacon or grease in your new lifestyle.

146. Instead of buying commercial granola mixes, which may contain up to 30 percent fat, try making your own. Mix together four cups dry oatmeal, three cups All-Bran, one teaspoon cinnamon, one cup orange juice, one teaspoon vanilla, one cup Bran Flakes, one cup golden raisins, a small peeled and chopped apple, half a teaspoon nutmeg, half a cup wheat germ, half a cup slivered almonds, and one teaspoon almond extract. Combine all ingredients except for raisins and bake in a nonstick pan for fifty minutes at 250 degrees. Add the raisins in the last ten minutes.

147. Potatoes are low in calories and fat and are extremely filling. The outside skin is a great source of fiber. Branch out and stuff your potatoes with all sorts of ethnic foods such as (1) Mexican style, stuffed with grilled onions and bell peppers, then top with nonfat plain yogurt; (2) Russian style, stuffed with a low-cal Beef Stroganoff; (3) Italian style, stuffed with ricotta cheese and spaghetti sauce; (4) Texas style, stuffed with lowfat chili and topped with Alpine Lace fat-free cheese and chopped green onion; (5) Greek style, stuffed with one tablespoon of feta cheese and two tablespoons of nonfat plain yogurt; and (6) Indian style, stuffed with lowfat curried chicken.

148. Other stuffed vegetables make for a nice way to decrease the meat content and increase vegetable content of the meal. Stuffed bell peppers and squashes seem to work best. Poblano peppers (which are very mild if you take out the seeds) make a nice base for a favorite lowfat meat loaf recipe.

149. When at a party, make a point to develop your conversations away from the food table. Stand across the room from the refresh-

ments if at all possible. If you watch other people stand there and snack, you may be tempted to do the same. If foods are placed in front of you on a table, try to relocate them.

150. Take the healthy eating message to others. This is the essence of the last step of recovery.

Be Prepared for Maintenance and Relapse

There are three main reasons people regain weight after dieting. First, many dieters falsely think that after the weight is gone they can have an eating heyday. I mentioned earlier in this book that if you go back to your old ways, you will also go back to your old weight. That is information you can bank on.

The focus of this book has been *lifestyle change*. By sticking to your weight-loss regimen for several months, you have actually been in training for your maintenance diet. By the time you are in the final phases of reaching your target weight, you will be losing weight at a snail's pace. Perhaps one pound per week, if you are lucky. Then to make that subtle switch from losing to maintaining, it will only require the manipulation of a few hundred calories per day. This does not constitute a major change in the way you are doing things. In fact, the maintenance plan should consist of the same types of foods, just in greater quantities and with a few additional and occasional food extravagances.

It only takes two hundred extra calories per day that you do not metabolize to cause a twenty-pound weight gain in one year's time. Many dieters will gain back as many as sixty or even eighty pounds in one year. You may tell yourself that this would never happen to you. If you have taken this book to heart, chances are it will not happen. But for dieters that go through a quick weight-loss program and then come off of it thinking they can now eat whatever they want, the old habits will cause them to return to their previous pre-diet weight.

A second reason dieters regain weight is because they are now burning fewer calories. It takes a 130 pound woman fewer calories to get around than a 180 pound woman. For the 180 pound person, is is like hauling a fifty-pound pack on her back, day in, day out. That burns a lot of calories! If you work on building those muscles, how-ever, you can usually offset many of these decreased, calorie-burning issues.

And third, for about six to twelve months after the weight has been lost, your metabolism may be slightly depressed. Your body is adjusting to its new weight. You are adjusting to the new you. Post-dieting metabolism usually pops back up after this pe-riod of latency, and if you can survive the first year after losing weight without gaining any or much of it back, you usually have it made.

YOUR MAINTENANCE DIET

Your maintenance diet should consist of the same lowfat foods (below 25 percent of the total calories as fat) as before. Just switch to a higher calorie level. You may want to plan your maintenance meals using food exchanges from pages 34–43) in the same way that you have planned your weight-loss diet. Since fat cells can be refilled with fat, it is essential that we should not return to high-fat foods after all the weight is lost.

This is a good time to increase your intake of pure calories, like complex carbohydrates. If you are already consuming two glasses of milk and six ounces of meat, you are certainly getting your protein requirement and then some. Set your sights on foods that provide nutrients and calories, not fat or additional protein.

Now let's look at a few red flags that should be your signals for taking stock of the situation and avoiding weight regain before it ever happens.

Red Flag Number 1: Are you changing your grocery shopping patterns?

Let's get honest on this one. I've done it myself. You are at the supermarket, you have done well on a diet, and you fall for the Christmas colored peanut M & M's. That starts the holiday binge, and you are not back in control for six months.

Does that sound familiar? Some people ask me if they will ever be able to have items like this in their home. I can't answer that question for you. Only you really know the answer. One question I have, though, is who are these specialty foods for? Who will eat them? Are they really required by other members of your household?

If we consider that for most of us food addiction and compulsive overeating has been a part of our past, it is also safe to say there is the possibility of falling back into old and comfortable ways. If you were an alcoholic, you would not go back and hang around bars after your recovery. Why do we put ourselves through this with food? If delicious but inappropriate food items are in the house, they will be eaten—perhaps by you. It is advisable to respect your new boundaries by rarely or never bringing high-cal, high-fat foods into the house.

Red Flag Number 2: Are you eating much larger portion sizes?

It is expected that you should eat larger portions when you are beginning to maintain your weight. But how much larger? It has been a long time since you have been at your ideal weight. Perhaps forever. You just don't have any frame of reference for what it takes to maintain this weight. You only know what you did in the past. But those days are gone forever. It is important to calculate how much you should be eating using the exchange lists at a calorie level suitable for maintenance. Your new calorie level should be approximately your weight in pounds times 12 to 14. In most cases, you will no longer desire the larger amounts of food, but improper food choices may pose a greater threat.

Watch for reinstigating family-style meals, seconds, and television snacking, since these may play a specific role in consuming larger portion sizes.

Red Flag Number 3: Are you going back to old recipes in greater frequency?

Those old high-fat chicken casserole recipes using sour cream and cream cheese should be in the distant past—forever. Your new lifestyle has too many wonderful new alternatives. Throw those recipes out for good and don't buy new recipe books that are unsympathetic to the cause.

Red Flag Number 4: Are you allowing yourself to eat differently because of new and different situations?

In 1992 at least 30 percent of my patients wondered about job security. In fact, many were in constant fear that their jobs might dry up in the next month. My advice was to live cautiously, taking risks and chances when they are more of a sure deal than a risk. Living under stressful conditions can only cause you trouble whether you are dieting or maintaining.

Many stressors in our world are uncontrollable. If you live in the San Francisco Bay area, you certainly cannot control earthquakes. If someone in your family (or yourself) becomes critically ill, you cannot control what will happen next. But if you have only enough money in the bank to cover two months of living expenses if your job were to end, this is probably in your control. I am convinced that we bring many of life's stressors on ourselves.

Nonetheless, when stress does come, try to be careful that your diet does not jump the tracks and try to compensate for a lifestyle that seems challenging or difficult in other areas.

Red Flag Number 5: Have your exercise habits changed?

Too many of us tend to punish our overeating by not exercising. All or none. I either diet (or do well with maintenance) and keep up my exercise, or I do nothing at all. Try to develop the mind-set that we are doing exercise for fun. Exercise should be a separate issue from food.

Researchers continually state that the main area most indicative of successful weight-loss maintenance is whether someone keeps up their exercise. This extra two hundred to four hundred calories per day that is burned up could be just the thing keeping you from gaining back at that twenty-pound-per-year rate.

Red Flag Number 6: Have you gained five pounds?

This should be the flashbulb that goes off in your head. Five pounds is as much as you should ever gain back. If this happens, you should temporarily back off of your schedule, take some time for yourself, and get back on track. This may mean cancelling a few social engagements or taking a few vacation days. You can jump-start yourself by emptying the house of trigger foods, replacing them with healthy food choices, and getting at least double exercise for a few days to help motivate you.

SUMMING IT UP

Here we are at the end of the book. I want to leave you with a summation of the essentials I believe are the cornerstones of permanent weight loss and weight control. Keep this list handy, and challenge yourself to see if you are fulfilling these requirements.

1. Weight loss takes a long time. I must set reasonable goals for myself and be happy for every success.

2. To lose weight, I must give up eating a high-fat diet—forever.

3. I should keep my fat intake below 25 percent of the total calories.

4. I know that I can't lose weight and keep it off until I exercise a minimum of two hours per week.

5. I know it is likely that I was once addicted to food. I further recognize that this addiction could be renewed if I am not vigilant about healthy habits and feelings.

6. I recognize that I need to learn how to choose foods and cook differently. The old ways and ingredients just won't do anymore.

7. I recognize that I am a whole person and that I should pay attention to all areas of my life and happiness.

8. I recognize that it will take about a year after I have lost my weight to fully stabilize and become accustomed to the new me.

All You Ever Wanted to Know about Poultry—and Then Some

For many of us, poultry of all types has taken over as the meat of choice in our attempt to decrease fat and caloric intake. But within the last several years many questions have arisen as to the chicken and poultry industry in general and the quality of product that reaches our shopping cart. Let's take a look at some facts and figures about poultry.

Poultry Facts and Figures

• Cholesterol levels for poultry range from seventy to ninety-five milligrams per 3.5 ounce serving. This is about the same amount as beef. However, it is lower in saturated fat than is the same amount of beef. Chicken liver contains over six hundred milligrams of cholesterol for that same 3.5 ounce serving, or about the same amount found in at least six greasy cheeseburgers.

• Duck, goose, and capon (see table page 58) are more fatty than chicken and beef and should be eaten less often.

• Oven baking a whole bird at a low temperature for a long period of time will remove more fat than any other method. You may leave the skin on for this process for a more moist final product. Just remember to avoid eating the skin when it is served.

• White meat of all varieties of poultry is lower in fat than dark meat. The white meat of turkey is the lowest fat of all poultry.

• By discarding the skin and trimming all visible fat from poultry parts, you may reduce the fat content by up to half.

• The meat from small chickens (broiler/fryers and Cornish game hens) is usually leaner than that from larger birds.

Poultry Q and A

Question: Is poultry lower in cholesterol than beef?

Answer: No. Cholesterol is not the same as saturated fat. In fact, all animal products contain about twenty to twenty-five milligrams of cholesterol per ounce no matter how lean it is otherwise. There is less saturated fat in poultry than there is even in the leanest cuts of beef or pork, however. And, since saturated fat turns into cholesterol in the human body, there is still reason to choose poultry as a major source of meat.

Question: Is ground turkey a better choice than ground beef?

Answer: That depends on whether or not the skin and fat was ground up with the lean portion of the turkey. A new super-lean ground beef on the market from Healthy Choice™ shows their product to contain 130 calories and 4 grams of fat for a 3.5 ounce serving of cooked ground beef. This is a lot leaner than many commercial ground turkey products. If you are buying turkey that is not packaged commercially, be sure you know what you are getting and whether your source of information concerning the product is reliable. Otherwise, one of the new, leaner ground beef products may be more desirable.

Question: Are yellow-skinned chickens less or more nutritious?

Answer: They are the same, nutrition-wise. The color of the skin depends on the feed that is given the bird. If the chicken is fed substances that have a lot of yellow color, such as marigold petals, then the skin and fat will take on a yellow appearance.

Question: What about game birds including quail, pheasant, squab, and guinea hen?

Answer: Almost all game (whether poultry or not) is leaner than its commercialized counterpart simply because animals in the wild don't get fat. (Maybe we should all move to the woods!) Calorie amounts are close to those of lean fish and range from 110 to 130 calories per 3.5-ounce cooked serving.

Question: Is chicken safe to eat, considering all the information out on salmonella contamination?

Answer: At least half (and possibly much more) of all raw chicken marketed in the United States is contaminated by salmonella or campylobacter. And at least 1500 to 2000 Americans die each year from this type of food poisoning. Six million others will become ill from salmonella or campylobacter poisoning. The good news is that these organisms can be killed with heat and their growth is inhibited by refrigeration. Poultry is safe if handled properly.

Safe Handling of Chicken

- Poultry must be cooked thoroughly, whether eaten at home or out. Juices should always run clear, not pink. If it is pink in a restaurant, send it back for more cooking. Cook to 180 degrees Fahrenheit if at home.

- Do not place raw chicken on a porous surface that cannot be thoroughly cleaned, such as wood.

- Do not let raw chicken touch any other foods that will be served raw, such as fruits, salads, or other vegetables.

- When barbecuing chicken, do not put cooked chicken back on the same plate that once carried the raw chicken. This might still carry germs.

- Thaw frozen poultry in the refrigerator. When in a hurry use the microwave and cook immediately.

- Make sure that leaking fluids from your poultry packages don't come in contact with lettuce and other products from the grocery store. Place packages of raw chicken in the extra plastic bags that are usually available at most meat counters.

- When marinating chicken, do so in the refrigerator rather than at room temperature where organisms may grow.

- Refrigerate raw poultry immediately, don't keep it refrigerated for more than two days. Cooked poultry can be safely refrigerated for up to four days.

- If stuffing a bird, do not let it stand at room temperature. Try making the stuffing ahead, chilling it, and then stuffing the bird prior to cooking. The stuffing should be cooked to 160 degrees Fahrenheit to eliminate contamination from poultry juices. After serving the dinner, remove the stuffing from the cavity and refrigerate separately.

Comparing Poultry Meats

Type of Food	Calories	Fat (g)	% Calories
Chicken (broiler/fryer)			
Breast, no skin	165	3.5	19
Wing, no skin	203	8.1	36
Drumstick, no skin	172	5.6	29
Thigh, no skin	209	10.8	47
Chicken (roasting)			
Light meat, no skin	153	4.1	24
Dark meat, no skin	178	8.8	44
Turkey			
Breast, no skin	135	0.7	5
Dark meat, no skin	186	7.0	34

High-fat Poultry

Chicken skin, amount eaten with one breast	112	10.0	81
Chicken thigh, with skin	247	15.5	56
Duck, all parts, no skin	201	11.2	50
Duck, all parts, with skin	337	28.4	76
Goose, all parts, no skin	238	12.7	48
Goose, all parts, with skin	305	21.9	65

Nutritional values always vary with individual cooking methods and genetically different animals. The above figures will usually be within 10 percent of the actual nutritional value.

The Story on Seafood

The seafood industry has practically been harpooned out of the water with nationwide allegations that fish is unfit to eat. Some reports show that nearly one in three samples of fish bought over a six month investigation was of poor quality when sent for laboratory testing. More specifically, the fish was bacteria-ridden and full of toxins. Nonetheless, unspoiled fish is still the best lowfat meat source. What can we trust with regard to seafood and how can we spot a wholesome seafood product?

Most of the contamination of seafood is bacterial. Large numbers of bacteria can decrease the overall quality and taste of fish, but if thoroughly cooked can be rendered harmless. Here are some tips on how you can show like a pro at the fish market.

1. Let your nose do the talking—never buy anything that smells "fishy." A slight seaweed or cucumber-like odor is expected, but a strong smell of fish or ammonia usually signifies that enough bacteria have multiplied on the surface to decrease the taste and texture.

2. Look for the flesh to be moist and shiny rather than dry and lack-luster. It should also bounce back when gently pressed.

3. If buying the whole fish rather than fillets, the fish should look as if it were right out of the water. The gills should be pink to even bright red rather than gray, brown, or green. The eyes should be bright, clear, and full instead of sunken and cloudy.

4. If fillets are piled high on a single layer of ice, naturally you want the ones closer to the bottom of the stack. The ones on top will have a greater bacterial growth because they are not being kept as cold.

5. Don't buy items containing cooked fish, such as seafood salads, that are displayed alongside raw fish. This is particularly dangerous because some of the bacteria from the raw fish may have slipped into the salad (often with a mayonnaise base). Since these already-cooked products will not be recooked, there is a particular threat of unchecked contamination.

6. Fresh fish brought home from the market should be stored in the coldest part of your refrigerator to help retard bacterial growth. Fish keeps longest in refrigerators that are kept at thirty-two to thirty-eight degrees Fahrenheit, yet many people have theirs at forty degrees or higher. To check the temperature in your unit, use a refrigerator thermometer. These are available at most supermarkets and hardware stores.

7. Try not to store fish more than two days if unfrozen. It spoils faster than either beef or poultry. The best method is to buy what you need and plan on cooking fish on market day.

8. In light of recent discoveries about the high degree of bacterial contamination of fish, it is preferable to heat fish at 450 degrees for about ten minutes for every inch of thickness. This is more effective at destroying bacteria than a 325 or 350 oven for thirty to forty minutes. Fish is fully cooked when the watery, translucent appearance becomes more opaque. When fully cooked, it flakes with a fork.

More Problems Than Bacteria

Proper food handling, storage, and cooking methods can easily handle seafood bacteria. Beyond this issue, though, is the problem with pollutants and contaminants from industrial residues. Among the most bothersome are PCBs, or polychlorinated biphenyls. They were actually banned in 1979 but continue to linger in our waterways into which they were once dumped. PCBs continue to show up in the tissues of salmon, swordfish, lake whitefish, and others. The greatest concern here is for pregnant women and their developing babies.

A second concern is the level of mercury found in fish. It is a poisonous metal released into the water by the burning of fuels and by industrial waste. It can accumulate in larger fish that live for many years, including tuna, shark, and swordfish. Again, most of the warnings are for pregnant women. And there is just not enough long-term data for us to know how adults are affected and at what levels.

Ultimately, this type of information does make us think about going back to beans and rice. Actually, the lower we eat on the food chain, the less likely the foods are to contain contaminants. I think of these high carbohydrate and higher calorie foods as the best choices for weight maintenance (when prepared in fat-free ways). But higher quality proteins may still give you an edge in the weight-loss game.

Most experts still agree that our fish supply is safe. Just be careful when making selections and in your cooking methods.

The Real Story on Ground Beef

The *Environmental Nutrition Newsletter* (May 1992) pointedly asks if the substance we often make into a meat loaf should be more correctly called ground beef or ground fat. This is a question of significance, since beef makes up to 44 percent of the total meat sales in the U.S., causing it to be the single largest source of fat in the American diet.

You are no doubt thinking, "But I only buy the leanest ground beef." Well, check these results provided by the National Livestock and Meat Board.

Translating % Lean Into % Fat

Labeling on ground beef is expressed as % lean by weight. But thinking of it in terms of % calories from fat is more revealing.

Ground beef labeled as:	Provides:
73% lean	79% percent calories from fat
80% lean	71% percent calories from fat
85% lean	64% percent calories from fat
90% lean	53% percent calories from fat
95% lean	34% percent calories from fat

Information provided by Eric Hentges, Ph.D., National Livestock and Meat Board, and *Environmental Nutrition,* May, 1992.

The problem we really face is not the lean part of the beef, but which beef parts are actually ground by individual grocers and then marketed as lean meat. Honest labeling is the real issue. Though reforms are on their way, the new labeling for beef and poultry has just been extended to May 1994.

The actual amount of fat in extra lean ground round varies depending on where it was purchased. Fat content varies from state to state and even from store to store. Have you ever noticed how the extra lean from one grocer seems to have a lot of fat that cooks out while another sticks to the bottom of the pan? Find out where the leanest ground beef can be found in your area. Lean ground round is no problem. Just make sure they do not grind in the surrounding fat to increase their margin of profit.

Alternatives to Ground Fat

It's not all bad news, hamburger lovers. Here are a few tips that may help:

- Choose lean round steaks or roasts and have the butcher trim all extra fat and make you your own special grind. If you can find a special on round steak, it costs no more.
- New lowfat products that substitute for grocery store ground beef are Lean Maker Superlean™ and Healthy Choice Extra Lean Ground Beef™, both of which contain no more than 30 percent of the calories as fat.

Low Calorie Recipes

CLASSIC CHEESECAKE

Nutritional Information
$1/8$-of-recipe serving:
Calories 103
Fat 1.8g
Protein 6g
Carbohydrates 23.7g
% fat 16
Cholesterol 0

Exchanges
$1/2$ Bread
1 Milk

32-ounce carton lowfat, vanilla-flavored yogurt
4 tablespoons granulated sugar
1 tablespoon cornstarch
1 tablespoon lemon juice
1 teaspoon vanilla
$1/2$ cup Egg Beaters (or 2 whole eggs)
Nonstick cooking spray

Prepare Basic Yogurt Cheese (page 227), substituting vanilla yogurt for plain. Use the entire carton of yogurt. Use nonstick cooking spray on an 8-inch pie pan or 7-inch springform pan. In a mixing bowl, combine the yogurt cheese with all remaining ingredients. Prepare Crumb Crust from Pineapple Cheesecake recipe (page 222), pour mixture into crust, and bake in a 325° preheated oven for 20 to 25 minutes in a pie pan or 40 to 45 minutes in a springform pan. Cool and refrigerate until serving. Add fresh strawberries to the top, if desired. Serves 8.

PINEAPPLE CHEESECAKE

Nutritional Information
1/8-of-pie serving:
Calories 105
Fat 1g
Protein 10g
Carbohydrates 15g
% fat 8
Cholesterol 20mg

Exchanges
1/2 Bread
1/2 Milk
1/2 Fruit

2 envelopes unflavored gelatin
1/4 cup sugar
1/4 teaspoon salt
1/2 cup unsweetened pineapple juice
1 cup lowfat milk
3 egg whites
8 ounces lowfat cottage cheese
1/2 cup crushed pineapple, drained
1 tablespoon lemon peel, grated
1/2 cup graham cracker crumbs
1 teaspoon vanilla
1 tablespoon diet margarine
3 tablespoons pineapple juice
1 tablespoon lemon juice
2 tablespoons sugar
3 tablespoons crushed pineapple, drained

In a saucepan, mix gelatin, 3/4 cup sugar, salt, 1/2 cup pineapple juice, milk, and 1 egg white. Cook over low heat until mixture thickens. Cool slightly, pour into blender. Add cottage cheese. Liquefy. Stir in pineapple and lemon peel. In a small bowl, combine graham cracker crumbs, vanilla, 3 tablespoons pineapple juice, lemon juice, and 2 tablespoons sugar. Mix and pack into a 9-inch pie plate. Pour in cheese mixture. Chill until firm, and top with remaining 3 tablespoons of drained pineapple. Serves 8.

CLASSIC BANANA SPLIT

Nutritional Information
Entire-recipe serving:
Calories 302
Fat 7g
Protein 7g
Carbohydrates 52g
% fat 21
Cholesterol 0

Exchanges
1 Bread
1 Milk
1 Fruit
1 Fat

⅓ cup chocolate ice milk
⅓ cup strawberry ice milk
½ small banana
1 tablespoon strawberry jam
1 tablespoon crushed pineapple
1 tablespoon walnuts, chopped

In a banana split dish, put ⅓-cup scoops of chocolate and strawberry ice milk. Slice the banana lengthwise, and place ½ on each side of the ice milk. Top the scoops of ice milk with the fruit toppers. Finish with the chopped nuts. Serves 1.

Sure it's a splurge—but only a 300-calorie splurge instead of 1,000 calories. Have this great dessert on some special occasion.

FRUIT SMOOTHIES

Nutritional Information
1-cup serving:
Calories 45
Fat 0
Protein 0
Carbohydrates 11.5g
% fat 0
Cholesterol 0

Exchanges
1 Fruit

1 cup fresh strawberries
1 small banana
1 teaspoon sugar
1–2 cups crushed ice and water
4 large, fresh strawberries

Combine all ingredients in a blender and mix until smooth. Pour equally into 4 glasses. Cut a strawberry partially in half (leaving the top intact) and wedge onto the side of the glass. Serve immediately. Serves 4.

Other fruits may be used instead of the strawberries. However, they are particularly low in calories.

NO-CHOLESTEROL BROWNIES

Nutritional Information
1-square serving:
Calories 105
Fat 4g
Protein 7.1g
Carbohydrates 10.1g
% fat 34
Cholesterol 0

Exchanges
1 Bread
1 Fat

¼ cup corn oil margarine
½ cup sugar
½ cup brown sugar, firmly packed
½ cup all-purpose flour
2 tablespoons unsweetened cocoa
2 egg whites
1 teaspoon vanilla extract
¼ cup walnuts, chopped
Nonstick cooking spray

Melt the margarine in a large bowl. Add all other ingredients except walnuts. Mix well. Stir in walnuts. Spread out batter evenly in an 8″x8″x2″ metal pan sprayed with nonstick cooking spray. Bake at 350° for 30 minutes or until just done. The middle portion should still be soft. Cool before cutting into 2-inch squares. Serves 16.

Any cookie recipe may be modified in a similar way as has been done with this one to yield a lower-fat, lower-calorie, lower-cholesterol product.

THANKSGIVING PUMPKIN PIE

Nutritional Information
1/10-of-recipe serving:
Calories 175
Fat 4.7g
Protein 12g
Carbohydrates 21.2g
% fat 24
Cholesterol 0

Exchanges
1 Bread
½ Milk
1 Fruit

½ cup Egg Beaters
1 16-ounce can pumpkin, solid-pack
¾ cup brown sugar, firmly packed
½ teaspoon salt
1 teaspoon ground cinnamon
½ teaspoon ground ginger
¼ teaspoon ground cloves
1 12-ounce can evaporated skim milk
1 9-inch deep-dish pastry piecrust

Combine all the ingredients, except the piecrust, in the order given. Mix until smooth. Pour into the 9-inch piecrust, and bake 15 minutes at 425°.

Reduce the temperature to 350°, and bake an additional 40 to 50 minutes or until a knife inserted in the center comes out clean. Serves 10.

SKINNY FRENCH FRIES

Nutritional Information
¹/₂-potato serving:
Calories 120
Fat 2g
Protein 2g
Carbohydrates 23g
% fat 15
Cholesterol 0

Exchanges
1¹/₂ Bread
¹/₂ Fat

2 large Idaho potatoes, unpeeled and cut in strips
PAM butter-flavored cooking spray
Seasoned salt, pepper, or Cajun seasoning mix

Wash and prepare the potatoes. Dry the surface of the potato strips by placing them on paper towels. Spray a nonstick cookie sheet with PAM. Spray the potatoes with PAM and then sprinkle with seasoning of choice (you might try shaking them in a clear plastic bag). Bake at 350° for 30 to 35 minutes until tender and golden brown. Turn occasionally with a spatula. Serves 4.

PARTY CHEESE BALL

Nutritional Information
¹/₁₀-of-the-recipe serving:
Calories 94
Fat 7.7g
Protein 4.4g
Carbohydrates 2g
% fat 73
Cholesterol 26mg

Exchanges
1 Meat
¹/₂ Fat

8 ounces Philadelphia light cream cheese
4 ounces mozzarella cheese, finely grated
2 teaspoons Worcestershire sauce
1 tablespoon sesame seeds
1 dash Tabasco sauce
3 tablespoons dried parsley flakes

Soften the cream cheese. Mix the first 5 ingredients. This can easily be accomplished in a food processor. After it has been mixed, roll into a ball shape. Spread parsley flakes on a plate, and then roll the cheese ball in the flakes to coat completely. Serves 10.

Serving Suggestions: This is a wonderful hors d'oeuvre for Christmas parties. Top the green ball with slices of red pimento or red bell pepper in the shape of a poinsettia.

Any cheese ball is extremely high in fat. If you

must have one, you can be moderate by eating only a small portion and by using these lower-fat cheeses.

BUTTERY POPCORN

Nutritional Information
3-cup serving:
Calories 108
Fat 1.5g
Protein 3.6g
Carbohydrates 21g
% fat 12
Cholesterol 0

Exchanges
1 Bread
½ Fat

½ cup uncooked popcorn
Butter-flavored cooking spray
Molly McButter
Mrs. Dash, no pepper.

Pop the popcorn in a microwave using a special plastic bowl designed for that purpose. Follow the directions that accompany the bowl. No oil should be necessary. When finished, spray with the cooking spray and sprinkle with Molly Mc-Butter and Mrs. Dash. Serves 3.

EASY TEXAS CHILI AND PINTOS

Nutritional Information
1-to-1½ cup serving:
Calories 198
Fat 3g
Protein 25.5g
Carbohydrates 17.2g
% fat 14
Cholesterol 25mg

Exchanges
1 Bread
1½ Meat
½ Vegetable

½ **pound dry pinto beans**
½ **pound dry kidney beans**
8 cups water
½ **teaspoon salt**
1 pound ground round
2 packages commercial chili seasoning mix
1 16-ounce can tomatoes, diced
1 large onion, diced
2 cloves garlic, diced
1 4-ounce can green chilis (optional)
1 bell pepper, diced
4 tablespoons Masa Harina (masa flour)
4 tablespoons water

Rinse the beans and soak in tap water for 2 to 3 hours until the beans plump. Boil the beans, water, and salt until they are soft. Brown the ground round. Add all remaining ingredients (except Masa Harina) and simmer 10 minutes. Combine the meat mixture with the beans. In a mixing bowl, combine the Masa Harina with 4 tablespoons of water to form a thick paste. Add to the chili and heat while stirring for 2 to 3 minutes. Serves 10.

RICOTTA VEGETABLE DIP

Nutritional Information
¹/₄-cup-of-dip serving:
Calories 67
Fat 2.5g
Protein 6.5g
Carbohydrates 4.8g
% fat 33
Cholesterol 7mg

Exchanges
¹/₂ Milk
¹/₂ Fat

8 ounces part-skim milk ricotta
8 ounces Basic Yogurt Cheese (p. 000)
2 tablespoons green olives, minced
¹/₄ cup carrots, minced
¹/₄ cup celery, minced
2 tablespoons pecans, minced
Carrots, celery, cucumbers, and yellow squash

Combine ricotta, yogurt cheese, olives, minced carrots, minced celery, and pecans. Mix well. Make dipping sticks out of the carrots and celery, and slice the cucumbers and squash. Arrange the dip and vegetables on a party tray. Serves 10.

BASIC YOGURT CHEESE

Nutritional Information
2-tablespoon serving:
Calories 24
Fat 0
Protein 2.3g
Carbohydrates 3.5g
% fat 0
Cholesterol 0

Exchanges
¹/₄ Milk

16 ounces nonfat plain yogurt
Yogurt funnel or 15″x15″ piece of cheesecloth

When using either a yogurt funnel or cheesecloth, simply place the yogurt into the meshed area and drain over a dish for approximately 24 hours. The watery whey will drain out of the yogurt, leaving a cheeselike substance similar in consistency to cream cheese. The longer the yogurt drains, the firmer it will become as more whey drains out. You can buy a yogurt funnel at many culinary cookshops. Serves 10.

Yogurt cheese is a wonderful lowfat alternative to any of the following:

Ricotta cheese (part-skim)	22 calories/tablespoon
Sour cream	30 calories/tablespoon
Cream cheese	52 calories/tablespoon
Mayonnaise	100 calories/tablespoon

By contrast yogurt cheese is 12 calories per tablespoon and has *no fat*. Yogurt cheese may be used as a substitute in cheese balls, spreads, dips, cheesecakes, etc.

THOUSAND ISLAND DRESSING

Nutritional Information
2-tablespoon serving:
Calories 34
Fat 1.2g
Protein 3g
Carbohydrates 3g
% fat 31
Cholesterol 14mg

Exchanges
1/2 Meat
1/2 Fat

1 1/2 cups low-cal cottage cheese
1/2 teaspoon dry mustard
2 tablespoons barbeque sauce
2 tablespoons lite mayonnaise
1 tablespoon sugar
2 tablespoons sweet pickle relish
2 hard-boiled eggs, chopped

Combine the cottage cheese, mustard, barbecue sauce, mayonnaise, and sugar in a blender. Liquefy. Stir in the pickle relish and eggs. Serves 20.

BLUE CHEESE DRESSING

Nutritional Information
1-tablespoon serving:
Calories 27
Fat 2g
Protein 1g
Carbohydrates 1.2g
% fat 67
Cholesterol 24mg

Exchanges
1/2 Fat

1 cup low-cal cottage cheese
1/2 cup lite mayonnaise
1/2 teaspoon salt
1/3 cup blue cheese, crumbled

Place the cottage cheese, mayonnaise, and salt in a blender. Liquefy. Stir in the blue cheese. Refrigerate several hours before using. Serves 32.

BRAN MUFFINS

Nutritional Information
1-muffin serving:
Calories 110
Fat 1.5g
Protein 6.3g
Carbohydrates 17.7g
% fat 12
Cholesterol 0

Exchanges
1 Bread
1 Fat

1 cup whole-wheat flour
1 cup bran flakes
1/4 cup Miller's Bran
2 tablespoons golden raisins
2 teaspoons baking powder
1 teaspoon baking soda
1 teaspoon cinnamon
Dash of nutmeg
3/4 cup evaporated skim milk
2 tablespoons corn oil
3/4 cup frozen apple-juice concentrate
1 teaspoon pure vanilla extract

In a mixing bowl, combine all the dry ingredients. Then add the liquids, mixing thoroughly. Fill muffin tins 2/3 full and bake for 20 minutes at 375 °F. Serves 16.

Each muffin contains approximately 2 grams of crude fiber.

CLUB SANDWICH

Nutritional Information
1-sandwich serving:
Calories 290
Fat 25.2g
Protein 25.5g
Carbohydrates 32.2g
%fat 18
Cholesterol 58mg

Exchanges
1 1/2 Bread
2 Meat
1/2 Milk
1 Fat

3 slices lite bread (40 calories/slice)
1 slice lite ham
1 slice turkey breast
1 slice Canadian bacon
1 slice lite processed cheese
2 thin slices tomato
Shredded lettuce and purple onion to taste
2 teaspoons lite mayonnaise

Toast the bread. Spread the mayonnaise on one side of the toast. Add in consecutive order: turkey breast, Canadian bacon, tomato, toast, ham, cheese, onion, and lettuce, and the final piece of toast. Serves 1.

This makes a special sandwich to serve guests. Stay on your diet even when there are special occasions.

LOW-CAL GRILLED CHEESE

Nutritional Information
1-sandwich serving:
Calories 150
Fat 4.7g
Protein 8g
Carbohydrates 18.9g
% fat 28
Cholesterol 5mg

Exchanges
1 Bread
½ Meat
1 Fat

2 slices lite bread (40 calories/slice)
1 slice lite processed cheese
2 teaspoons diet margarine

Spread margarine evenly over one side of each slice of bread. Place cheese in the middle. Heat on a grill, griddle, or skillet until browned on each side. Cheese in the center should be completely melted. Serves 1.

Regular, high-fat grilled cheese sandwiches are about 400–500 calories per sandwich.

VEGETARIAN VEGETABLE SOUP

Nutritional Information
2-cup serving:
Calories 50
Fat 0.5g
Protein 2g
Carbohydrates 9.2g
% fat 10
Cholesterol 0

Exchanges
½ Bread
1 Vegetable

1 teaspoon olive oil
1 medium onion, chopped
3 stalks celery, cut lengthwise
1 medium bell pepper, chopped
4 cups water
4 bouillon cubes
2 16-ounce cans diced tomatoes
3 medium potatoes, cut into large chunks
Spices to taste: salt, pepper, basil, thyme, bay leaf,
    coriander, oregano, and garlic powder

Sauté the onion, celery, and bell pepper in the olive oil in a large Dutch oven. Add the other ingredients and simmer until softened. Serves 6.

SPINACH QUICHE

Nutritional Information
1/6 of pie serving:
Calories 192.5
Fat 9.5g
Protein 10.8g
Carbohydrates 15.9g
% fat 44
Cholesterol 5mg

Exchanges
1 Bread
1 1/2 Meat
1 Vegetable
1 Fat

1 pre-prepared piecrust
1 10-ounce package frozen spinach
1 clove garlic, minced
1 cup Egg Beaters
1 cup reconstituted, evaporated skim milk
1/3 cup Parmesan cheese
2 tablespoons Romano cheese
1 teaspoon dried basil
1/2 teaspoon salt
1/8 teaspoon cayenne pepper

Bake the piecrust for 5 minutes. In a medium bowl, combine eggs, milk, cheeses, basil, salt, and pepper and mix thoroughly. Add the spinach and garlic. Pour spinach and egg mixture into the piecrust, and bake for 1 hour at 325°. Let the quiche cool and set for 10 minutes before serving. Serves 6.

Who says quiche must be made from whole eggs and cream? Try this delightful lowfat rendition of a traditional favorite.

HAMBURGER HASH

Nutritional Information
1/4 of recipe:
Calories 270
Fat 8g
Protein 22g
Carbohydrates 28g
% fat 27
Cholesterol 57

Exchanges
3 Meat
1 1/2 Starch
1 Vegetable

3/4 pound lean ground beef
1/2 cup frozen chopped onion
1/2 teaspoon bottled minced garlic *or*
    1/8 teaspoon garlic powder
1 large potato
1/2 cup cracked wheat
1/2 cup frozen chopped green pepper
2 teaspoons instant beef bouillon granules
3/4 teaspoon dried thyme, crushed
1/4 teaspoon pepper
1 1/2 cups water
1 large tomato

Cracked wheat adds special flavor and extra nutrition to this old standby.

Break ground meat into large pieces while adding it to a large skillet. Add frozen onion and garlic. Cook meat, onion, and garlic over high heat till meat is brown and onion is tender. Drain off fat.

While the meat is cooking, dice the *unpeeled* potato. Add potato to skillet, along with cracked wheat, frozen green pepper, bouillon granules, thyme, and pepper. Stir in water. Bring to boiling, then reduce heat. Cover and simmer for 15 minutes or till potatoes and cracked wheat are tender.

While meat mixture is cooking, cut the tomato into 8 wedges. Garnish meat mixture with tomato wedges. Makes 4 servings.

SWEDISH MEATBALLS

Nutritional Information
¹/₈ **recipe or about**
6–8-meatball serving:
Calories 215
Fat 8.1g
Protein 26g
Carbohydrates 9g
% fat 41.8
Cholesterol 72mg

Exchanges
3 Meat

1¹/₂ **pounds very lean ground beef**
2 **egg whites**
1 **tablespoon dry minced onion**
1 **tablespoon parsley, chopped or dry**
1¹/₂ **teaspoons salt**
1 **teaspoon nutmeg**
¹/₄ **teaspoon pepper**
¹/₄ **cup skim milk**
2 **cups skim milk**
4 **stalks celery, diced**
2 **beef bouillon cubes**
¹/₄ **teaspoon pepper**
1¹/₂ **tablespoon flour**

Combine the beef, egg, onion, parsley, 1¹/₂ teaspoons salt, nutmeg, ¹/₄ teaspoon pepper, and ¹/₄ cup milk. Shape into small balls. Broil. In a large saucepan, combine the 2 cups milk, celery, salt, pepper, and flour. Stir until the flour is dissolved. Heat until the sauce thickens, stirring constantly.

Add the meatballs. Simmer 15 minutes. Add water if necessary. Serves 8.

This recipe makes a wonderful party meatball that is lower in calories and fat than many others.

CHICKEN ENCHILADAS VERDES

Nutritional Information
2-enchilada serving:
Calories 250
Fat 4.4g
Protein 16.6g
Carbohydrates 37.2g
% fat 16
Cholesterol 0

Exchanges
1 3/4 Bread
1 Meat
1/10 Milk
1/10 Vegetable
1 1/3 Fat

2 cups cooked chicken, chopped (remove all skin and visible fat)
2 green onions, chopped
1/8 teaspoon garlic powder
10 corn tortillas
1 cup chicken broth, defatted
1/2 cup nonfat yogurt
2 teaspoons skim milk
Thinly sliced onion
Salsa verde (below)

Make salsa verde. Combine chicken, green onions, garlic powder, and 3 tablespoons salsa verde. Mix well. Heat 1/4 cup chicken broth in small skillet, until hot. Slip 1 tortilla into skillet, cook until softened (or soften tortillas in microwave). Drain on paper towel. Repeat with remaining tortillas, adding additional chicken broth every 3 to 4 tortillas or as needed. Fill each tortilla with 3 tablespoons of chicken mixture; roll up. Fill all tortillas and arrange seam-side down, in a single layer in shallow baking dish. Pour salsa verde over tortillas. Bake until sauce is bubbly, about 20 minutes in 350° oven. Mix yogurt and skim milk and spoon over enchiladas. Top with onion slices. Serves 5.

SALSA VERDE (GREEN SAUCE)

Nutritional Information
1-tablespoon serving:
Calories 6
Fat 0g
Protein 0.1g
Carbohydrates 1.4g
% fat 2
Cholesterol 0

Exchanges
1/8 Vegetable

1 small onion
1 medium jalapeno, stemmed and chopped
1 tablespoon cilantro, chopped
1 small garlic clove, chopped
1 pound fresh tomatillos

Combine onion, jalapeno, cilantro, tomatillos and garlic in blender.

BLACKENED ORANGE ROUGHY

Nutritional Information
4-ounce serving:
Calories 190
Fat 3.7g
Protein 32g
Carbohydrates 7.8g
% fat 16
Cholesterol 75mg

Exchanges
4 Meat
1 Fat

20-ounces orange roughy fillets, raw
Nonstick butter-flavored cooking spray
1 1/2 tablespoons butter (or oil)
McCormick's blackened redfish mix (or something similar in another brand)
2 fresh lemons

Sprinkle fillets with seasoning mix. Spray a heavy skillet (such as copper lined with stainless steel) with butter-flavored nonstick cooking spray, and place on rangetop over medium heat. Melt butter in pan. Place fillets in hot skillet and cook 3 to 5 minutes on each side until fish is flaky. Turn off pan, sprinkle with fresh lemon juice. Serve immediately with more lemon juice, brown rice pilaf, and a vegetable. Serves 4.

BROWN RICE PILAF

Nutritional Information
1/2-cup serving:
Calories 104
Fat 0.7g
Protein 5g
Carbohydrates 18.7g
% fat 6
Cholesterol 0

Exchanges
1 Bread
1/4 Vegetable
1/4 Fat

2 cups brown rice
2 1/2 cups chicken stock, defatted
1 tablespoon diet margarine
1/4 teaspoon garlic powder
Dash of white pepper
Dash of black pepper
1/4 cup green pepper, chopped
1/4 cup onion, chopped
1/4 cup celery, chopped
2 tablespoons pimiento
Nonstick cooking spray

Spray baking dish with a nonstick cooking spray. Add rice to baking dish. Combine chicken stock, margarine, garlic powder, and peppers. Add to rice. Stir in green pepper, onion, celery, and pimiento. Cover with aluminum foil. Bake in 350° preheated oven for 50 minutes. Serves 8.

Combine onion, jalapeno, cilantro, tomatilles and garlic in blender.

SUMMARY WEIGHT-LOSS GRAPH

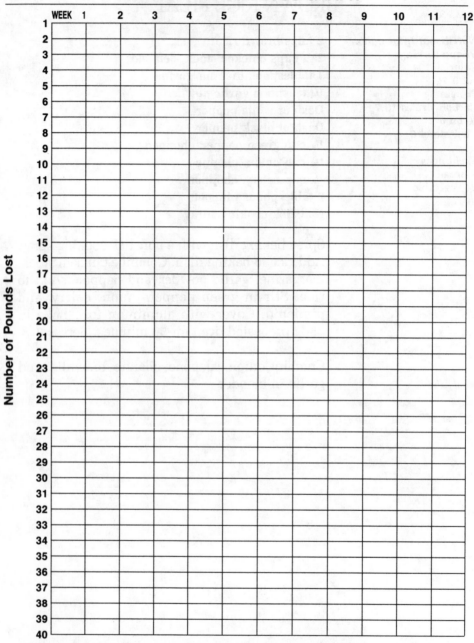

Number of Pounds Lost

WEEK 1 2 3 4 5 6 7 8 9 10 11 12

You can use the Summary Weight-Loss Graph above to record your weight loss in two different ways. You can either record the number of pounds you lose each week (see the dotted line in the sample graph) or you can see the total number of pounds you lose as you progress through the Twelve Week Weight-Loss Diet Plan (see the solid line in the sample graph). To see your total weight loss, record in the first column the number of pounds you lose the first week. Then move to right for the second week and count down the number of pounds you lose that week.

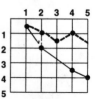

Notes

1. *Publisher's Weekly*, 1990.

2. Edwin Bierman, "Contemporary Management of the Overweight Patient," Opinion Leaders' Symposium Proceedings, June 15, 1991, Tempe, AZ.

3. Laura Pawlak, *Life Without Diets* (self-published, 1991).

4. F. Minirth, P. Meier, R. Hemfelt, and S. Sneed, *Love Hunger: Recovery from Food Addiction,* (Nashville, Tenn.: Thomas Nelson Publishers, 1990), p. 130.

5. F. Minirth, P. Meier, *Love Is a Choice,* (Nashville: Thomas Nelson, 1989).

6. Robert Hemfelt, Love Hunger Seminar, Austin, Texas.

ABOUT THE AUTHOR

Dr. Sharon Sneed is a registered dietitian and a practicing nutritional consultant. She has been an assistant professor at the Medical University of South Carolina and a postdoctoral fellow at the University of California at Berkeley. She has written and coauthored more than a dozen research articles and books, including *Love Hunger Weight-Loss Workbook* and *Love Hunger: Recovery from Food Addiction*.